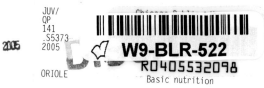
DATE DUE

Eating Right
An Introduction to Human Nutrition

Basic Nutrition

Nutrition and Eating Disorders

Nutrition for Sports and Exercise

Nutrition and Weight Management

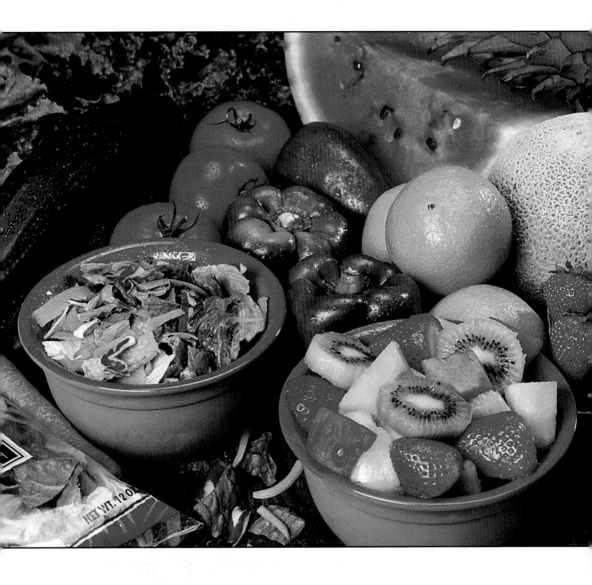

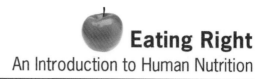

Eating Right

An Introduction to Human Nutrition

Basic Nutrition

Lori A. Smolin, Ph.D.
Mary B. Grosvenor, M.S., R.D.

Preface: Lori A. Smolin, Ph.D. and
Mary B. Grosvenor, M.S., R.D.

Introduction:
Richard J. Deckelbaum, MD, CM, FRCP(C)
Columbia University

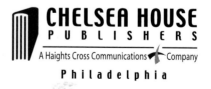

CHELSEA HOUSE

PUBLISHERS

A Haights Cross Communications Company

Philadelphia

Frontispiece: Proper nutrition is essential for a long and healthy life. Fruits and vegetables that are high in nutrients and low in fat are especially good choices for a healthful diet.

CHELSEA HOUSE PUBLISHERS
VP, New Product Development Sally Cheney
Director of Production Kim Shinners
Creative Manager Takeshi Takahashi
Manufacturing Manager Diann Grasse

Staff for BASIC NUTRITION
Executive Editor Tara Koellhoffer
Editor Beth Reger
Production Editor Megan Emery
Photo Editor Sarah Bloom
Series & Cover Designer Terry Mallon
Layout 21st Century Publishing and Communications, Inc.

A Haights Cross Communications  Company

www.chelseahouse.com

9 8 7 6 5 4 3 2

Library of Congress Cataloging-in-Publication Data

Smolin, Lori A.
   Basic nutrition/Lori A. Smolin, and Mary B. Grosvenor.
      p. cm.—(Eating right)
Includes bibliographical references and index.
   ISBN 0-7910-7850-7 (hardcover)—ISBN 0-7910-8015-3 (pbk.)
   1. Nutrition. I. Grosvenor, Mary B. II. Title. III. Series.
QP141.S5373 2004
613.2—dc22
                                        2004002745

All links and web addresses were checked and verified to be correct at the time of publication. Because of the dynamic nature of the web, some addresses and links may have changed since publication and may no longer be valid.

About the Authors

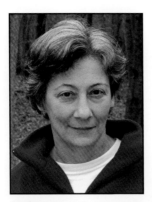

Lori A. Smolin, Ph.D. Lori Smolin received her B.S. degree from Cornell University, where she studied human nutrition and food science. She received her doctorate from the University of Wisconsin at Madison. Her doctoral research focused on B vitamins, homocysteine accumulation, and genetic defects in homocysteine metabolism. She completed postdoctoral training both at the Harbor–UCLA Medical Center, where she studied human obesity, and at the University of California at San Diego, where she studied genetic defects in amino acid metabolism. She has published in these areas in peer-reviewed journals. She and Mary Grosvenor are coauthors for two well-respected college-level nutrition textbooks and contributing authors for a middle school text. Dr. Smolin is currently at the University of Connecticut, where she teaches both in the Department of Nutritional Sciences and in the Department of Molecular and Cell Biology. Courses she has taught include introductory nutrition, lifecycle nutrition, food preparation, nutritional biochemistry, general biochemistry, and introductory biology.

Mary B. Grosvenor, M.S., R.D. Mary Grosvenor received her B.A. degree in English from Georgetown University and her M.S. in nutrition sciences from the University of California at Davis. She is a registered dietitian with experience in public health, clinical nutrition, and nutrition research. She has published in peer-reviewed journals in the areas of nutrition and cancer and methods of assessing dietary intake. She and Lori Smolin are the coauthors for two well-respected college-level nutrition textbooks and contributing authors for a middle school text. She has taught introductory nutrition at the community college level and currently lives with her family in a small town in Colorado. She is continuing her teaching and writing career and is still involved in nutrition research via the electronic superhighway.

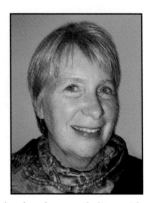

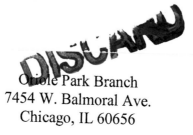

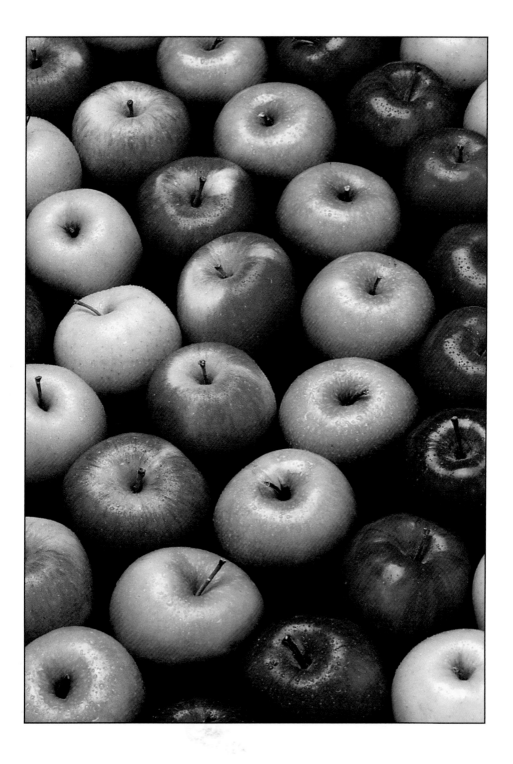

Contents Overview

Detailed Contents

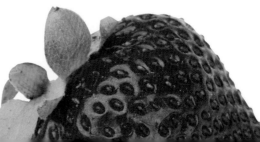

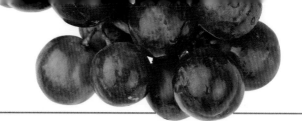

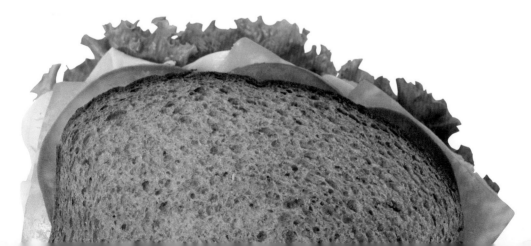

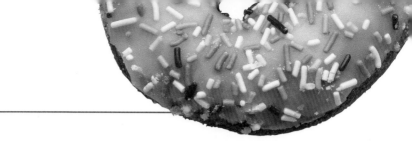

CHAPTER 9 CHOOSING A HEALTHY DIET ... 132

Preface

Lori A. Smolin, Ph.D.
Mary B. Grosvenor, M.S., R.D.

Fifty years ago we got our nutrition guidance from our mothers and grandmothers—eat your carrots, they are good for your eyes; don't eat too many potatoes, they'll make you fat; be sure to get plenty of roughage so your bowels move. Today, everyone has some advice—take a vitamin supplement to optimize your health; don't eat fish with cabbage because you won't be able to digest them together; you can't stay healthy on a vegetarian diet. Nutrition is one of those topics about which all people seem to think they know something or at least have an opinion. Whether it is the clerk in your local health food store recommending that you buy supplements or the woman behind you in line at the grocery store raving about the latest low-carbohydrate diet—everyone is ready to offer you nutritional advice. How do you know what to believe or, even more importantly, what to do?

Our purpose in writing these books is to help you answer these questions. As authors, we are students of nutrition. We enjoy studying and learning the hows and whys of each nutrient and other components of our diets. However, despite our enthusiasm about the science of nutrition, we recognize that not everyone loves science or shares this enthusiasm. On the other hand, everyone loves certain foods and wants to stay healthy. In response to this, we have written these books in a way that makes the science you need to understand as palatable as the foods you love. Once you understand the basics, you can apply them to your everyday choices regarding nutrition and health. We have developed one book that includes all the basic nutrition information you need to choose a healthy diet and three others that cover topics that are of special concern to many: weight management, exercise, and eating disorders.

Our goal is not to tell you to stop eating potato chips and candy bars, to give up fast food, or to always eat your vegetables. Instead, it is to provide you with the information you need to make informed choices about your diet. We hope you will recognize that potato chips and candy are not poison, but should only be eaten as occasional treats. We hope you will decide for yourself that fast food is something you can indulge in every now and then, but is not a good choice everyday. We hope you will recognize that although you should eat your vegetables, not everyone always does, so you should do your best to try new vegetables and fruits and eat them as often as possible. These books take the science of nutrition out of the classroom and allow you to apply this information to the choices you make about foods, exercise, dietary supplements, and other lifestyle choices that are important to your health. We hope the knowledge on these pages will help you choose a healthy diet while allowing you to enjoy the diversity of flavors, textures, and tastes that food provides and the meanings that food holds in our society. When you eat a healthy diet, you will feel good in the short term and enjoy health benefits in the long term. We can't personally evaluate your each and every meal, so we hope these books give you the tools to make your own nutritious choices.

This first book in the series EATING RIGHT: AN INTRODUCTION TO HUMAN NUTRITION is intended to establish the basics of food as fuel and how your body uses food to drive its processes. We discuss the six classes of nutrients, how each is broken down and used by the body, and how much of each an individual needs. We also provide some guidance to choosing a healthy diet.

Lori A. Smolin, Ph.D.
Mary B. Grosvenor, M.S., R.D.

Introduction

Richard J. Deckelbaum, MD, CM, FRCP(C)
Robert R. Williams Professor of Nutrition
Director, Institute of Human Nutrition
College of Physicians and Surgeons of Columbia University

Nutrition is a major factor in optimizing health and performance
at every age through the life cycle. While almost everyone recognizes
the devastating effects of severe undernutrition, often captured on
television during famines in underdeveloped parts of the world,
far fewer people recognize the problem of overnutrition that leads
to overweight and obesity. Even fewer are aware of the dangers
of "hidden malnutrition" associated with inadequate intake of
important vitamins and minerals. Unfortunately, there is also an
overabundance of inaccurate and misleading nutrition advice
being presented through media and books that makes it difficult for
teenagers and young adults to decide for themselves what really is
"optimal nutrition." This series, EATING RIGHT: AN INTRODUCTION TO
HUMAN NUTRITION, provides accurate information to help people
of all ages, and particularly young people, to acquire the needed
tools and knowledge to integrate good nutrition as part of a healthy
lifestyle. Each book in the series will be a comprehensive study in a
different area of nutrition and its applications. The series will stress
on many levels how healthy food choices affect the ability of people
to develop, learn, and be more successful in sports, work, and in
passing on good health to their families.

Beginning early in life, proper nutrition has major impacts. In
childhood, good nutrition is important not only in allowing normal
physical growth, but also in brain development and the ability to
acquire new knowledge, both in and out of school. For example,
proper dietary intake of iron is critical for preventing anemia, but
just as important, it also ensures the ability to learn in the classroom
and to be successful in sports or other spheres relating to physical
activity. Given the major contribution of sports and exercise in

improving health, it is easy to understand that nutrition truly is a partner with physical activity in promoting good health and better life outcomes.

Going into the adolescent years, many teenagers succumb to the dangers of fad diets—for example, undereating or alternatively overeating. Teens may not realize the impact of poor food choices upon their health, and, especially for girls, the risk that improper intake of vitamins and minerals will adversely impact their future families is very much underappreciated. As people mature into adults, nutritional practices have a major role in increasing or preventing the risk of major diseases such as stroke, heart attacks, and even a number of cancers. Thus, proper nutrition is an easy and cost-effective approach to achieving better growth and development, and later in markedly diminishing the chance of contracting many diseases.

Optimizing nutrition not only helps individuals but also has a major impact upon decreasing suffering and economic costs in families, communities, and nations. In the 21st century, individuals and populations will need to focus on at least three key areas. First, in promoting healthy lifestyles, nutrition needs to include a heavy concentration on diet and physical activity. Second, nutrition programs must focus on the realization that it is more important to work toward prevention rather than cure. Many of the early successes in nutrition focus on using nutrition as a treatment. We now know that improvement in nutritional status, which can easily be achieved, will have much more impact on preventing disease before it happens. Third, nutrition fits very well within the life cycle model. We know now that females who are healthy and fit *before* pregnancy are more likely to produce healthy babies and consequently healthy children. Conversely, women who have deficiencies of certain vitamins or unhealthy weights before pregnancy are more likely to have babies and children with significant health problems.

Developing countries now share the worldwide obesity epidemic. This series will help in the understanding that being overweight or obese not only changes physical appearance but also has a number of hidden dangers. For example, overweight and obesity are linked closely to rapid development of cardiovascular disease, type 2 diabetes, respiratory illnesses, and even liver disease and certain lung diseases. This "epidemic" must be fought by combined strategies using diet and physical activity. While many people today are striving to create more healthy lifestyles, they are unsure of how they should proceed. We feel that the books in this series will address these issues and provide the springboards for further thought and consideration about healthy eating.

Beginning with this first book in this series, EATING RIGHT: AN INTRODUCTION TO HUMAN NUTRITION, three more books will follow (*Nutrition for Sports and Exercise, Nutrition and Eating Disorders, Nutrition and Weight Management*). Thus, this first book presents the "nuts and bolts" needed to understand the "why's" of proper nutrition. This book, together with later editions in the series, will target specific areas to help readers achieve better outcomes for themselves and their families. With the knowledge to be gained through this series, we hope that each reader will be able to enhance his/her commitment to providing a better life for himself/herself and community.

Richard J. Deckelbaum, MD, CM, FRCP(C)
Robert R. Williams Professor of Nutrition
Director, Institute of Human Nutrition
College of Physicians and Surgeons
of Columbia University

1

What Is Nutrition?

Nutrition is the study of all of the interactions that occur between people and food. It involves understanding which **nutrients** we need, where to find them in food, how they are used by our bodies, and the impact they have on our health. It also has to consider the other factors, such as society, culture, economics, and technology, which are involved in obtaining and choosing the foods we eat.

WE GET NUTRIENTS FROM FOOD

We don't eat individual nutrients, we eat foods. When we choose the right combination of foods, our diet provides all of the nutrients we need to stay healthy. If we choose a poor combination of foods, we may be missing out on some **essential nutrients**. Choosing a diet that provides all of the essential nutrients can be challenging because we eat for many reasons other than to obtain nutrients. We eat because we see or smell a tempting food; because it's lunchtime; because we're at a party; because we are sad or happy; because it's Thanksgiving, Christmas, or Passover; and for a multitude of other reasons. In order to meet nutrient needs, we must understand what these needs are and how to choose a diet that provides them.

The Nutrients in Food

There are over 40 nutrients that are essential to human life. We need to consume these essential nutrients in our diets because they cannot be made by our bodies or they cannot be made in large enough amounts to optimize health. Different foods contain different nutrients in varying amounts and combinations. For example, beef, chicken, and fish provide protein, vitamin B_6, and iron; bread, rice, and pasta provide carbohydrate, folic acid, and niacin; fruits and vegetables provide carbohydrate, fiber, vitamin A, and vitamin C; and vegetable oils provide fat and vitamin E. In addition to the nutrients found naturally in foods, many foods have nutrients added to them to replace losses that occur during cooking and processing or to supplement the diet. Dietary supplements are also a source of nutrients. Although most people can meet their nutrient needs without them, supplements can be useful for maintaining health and preventing deficiencies.

What Do Nutrients Do?

Nutrients provide three basic functions in the body. Some nutrients provide energy, some provide structure, and some help to regulate the processes that keep us alive. Each nutrient performs one or more

---

FACT BOX 1.1

Who Checks Supplements for Safety?

According to the Dietary Supplement Health and Education Act of 1994, supplement manufacturers are responsible for ensuring that supplements are safe. The Food and Drug Administration (FDA) is only involved after the product is on the market. The FDA collects information about suspected problems with dietary supplements and has the authority to remove products from the market if it can prove that the product carries significant risk.

of these functions, and all nutrients together are needed for growth, to maintain and repair the body, and to allow us to reproduce.

Energy

Food provides the body with the energy or fuel it needs to stay alive, move, and grow. This energy keeps your heart pumping, your lungs inhaling, and your body warm. It is also used to keep your stomach churning and your muscles working. Carbohydrates, lipids, and proteins are the only nutrients that provide energy to the body; they are referred to as the energy-yielding nutrients. The energy used by the body is measured in **Calories** or **kilocalories** (abbreviated as kcalories or kcals) or in **kilojoules** (abbreviated as kjoules or kJs). When spelled with a lowercase "c," the term "**calorie**" is technically 1/1,000 of a kilocalorie. Each gram of carbohydrate we eat provides the body with 4 Calories. A gram of protein also provides 4 Calories; a gram of fat provides 9 Calories, more than twice the Calories of carbohydrate or protein. For this reason, foods that are high in fat are high in calories. Alcohol can also provide energy in the diet— 7 Calories per gram, but it is not considered a nutrient because it is not needed by the body.

If you eat more calories than you use, your body will store the extra energy mostly as body fat. When you consume the same number of calories as you use, your body weight remains the same. If you eat fewer than you use, your body will use its stored energy to fuel itself and you will lose weight.

Structure

Nutrients help form body structures. For example, the minerals calcium and phosphorus make our bones and teeth hard. Protein forms the structure of our muscles and lipids are the major component of our body fat. Water is a structural nutrient because it plumps up the cells. The body is more than 60% water.

Regulation

Nutrients are also important regulators of body functions. All of the processes that occur in our bodies, from the breakdown of carbohydrate and fat to provide energy, to the building of bone and muscle to form body structures, must be regulated for the body to function normally. For instance, the chemical reactions that maintain body temperature at 98.6°F (37°C) must be regulated or body temperature will rise above or fall below the healthy range. Many different nutrients are important in regulating **homeostasis** in the body. Carbohydrates help to label proteins that must be removed from the blood. Water helps to regulate body temperature. Lipids are needed to make regulatory molecules called **hormones**, and certain protein molecules, vitamins, and minerals help to regulate the rate of chemical reactions within the body.

Getting Nutrients to Your Cells

The food we eat must be digested and the nutrients must be absorbed for them to provide the body with the nourishment it needs. **Digestion** breaks food into small molecules and **absorption** brings these substances into the body, where they are transported to the cells.

The digestive system is responsible for the digestion and absorption of food (Figure 1.1). The main part of this system is the gastrointestinal tract, also called the GI tract. This hollow tube starts at the mouth. From there, food passes down the esophagus into the stomach and then on to the small intestine. Rhythmic contractions of the smooth muscles lining the GI tract help mix food and propel it along. Substances, such as **mucus** and **enzymes**, are secreted into the GI tract to help with the movement and digestion of food. The digestive system also secretes hormones into the blood that help regulate GI activity. Most of the digestion and absorption of nutrients occurs in the small intestine. Absorbed nutrients are transported in the blood to the cells. Anything that is not absorbed passes into the large intestine. Here, some nutrients can be absorbed and wastes are prepared for elimination.

How Your Body Uses Nutrients

Once inside body cells, carbohydrates, lipids, and proteins are involved in chemical reactions that allow them to be used for

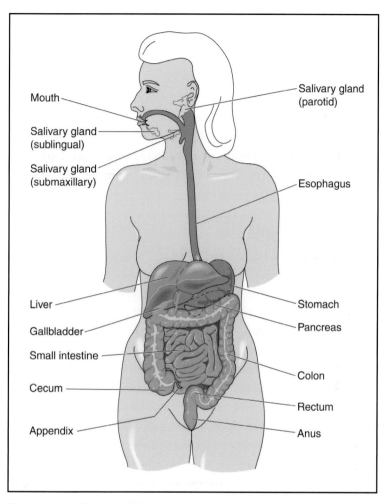

Figure 1.1 The digestive system consists of the gastrointestinal (GI) tract and accessory organs that aid digestion.

energy or to build other substances that are needed by the human body. The sum of the chemical reactions that occur inside body cells is called **metabolism**. The chemical reactions of metabolism can synthesize the molecules needed to form body structures such as muscles, nerves, and bones. The reactions of metabolism also break down carbohydrates, lipids, and proteins to yield energy in the form of **ATP (adenosine triphosphate)**. ATP is a molecule that is used by cells as an energy source to do work, such as to pump blood, contract muscles, or synthesize new body tissue.

THE SIX CLASSES OF NUTRIENTS

The nutrients we need come from six different classes: carbohydrate, lipid, protein, water, vitamins, and minerals. Each class, with the exception of water, contains a variety of different molecules that are used by the body in different ways. Some classes of nutrients are

---

FACT BOX 1.2

Bacteria in Your Intestine

Did you know that your large intestine is home to several hundred species of bacteria? You provide them with a nice warm home with lots of food and they do you some favors in return—if they are the right kind. These "good" bacteria improve the digestion and absorption of essential nutrients; synthesize some vitamins; and metabolize harmful substances, such as ammonia, thus reducing levels in the blood. They are important for intestinal immune function, proper growth of cells in the large intestine, and optimal intestinal motility and transit time. A healthy population of intestinal bacteria may also help prevent constipation, flatulence, and gastric acidity. However, if the wrong bacteria take over, the result could be diarrhea, infections, and perhaps an increased risk of cancer.

How can you make sure the right bacteria are growing in your gut? One way is to eat the bacteria. This is referred to as probiotic therapy. Live bacteria are found in foods such as yogurt and acidophilus milk and can be purchased as bottled suspensions or tablets. One problem with probiotic therapy is that the bacteria are washed out of the colon if you stop eating them. A second approach that can modify the bacteria in your gut is to consume foods or other substances that encourage the growth of particular types of bacteria. Substances that pass undigested into the large intestine and serve as food for these bacteria are called prebiotics. Prebiotics are sold as dietary supplements—but don't run to the store just yet. For most of us, eating a nutritious diet supports a healthy population of intestinal bacteria. Our understanding of how probiotics and prebiotics can be used to treat disease and promote health is still in its early stages.

needed in relatively large amounts whereas others meet needs when tiny amounts are consumed. Carbohydrate, lipid, protein, and water are often referred to as **macronutrients** because they are required in the diet in relatively large amounts. Vitamins and minerals are referred to as **micronutrients** because they are needed only in small amounts.

Carbohydrate

Carbohydrate includes **sugars**, **starches**, and **fibers**. Sugars are the simplest form of carbohydrate. They taste sweet and are found in fruit, milk, and added sugars like honey and table sugar. Starches are made of multiple sugar units linked together. They do not taste sweet and are found in cereals, grains, and starchy vegetables like potatoes. Starches and sugars are good sources of energy in the diet. Most fibers are also carbohydrates. Good sources of fiber include whole grains, legumes, fruits, and vegetables. Fiber provides little energy to the body because it cannot be digested or absorbed. It is, however, important for the health of the digestive tract.

Lipids

Lipids are commonly called fats. Fat is a concentrated source of energy. Most of the fat in our diet and in our bodies is in the form of **triglycerides**. Each triglyceride contains three **fatty acids**. Fatty acids are basically chains of carbon atoms. Depending on how these carbons are linked together, fats are classified as either **saturated** or **unsaturated**. Saturated fats are found mostly in animal products such as meat, milk, and butter. Unsaturated fats in our diets come from vegetable oils. Small amounts of certain unsaturated fatty acids are essential in the diet. **Cholesterol** is another type of fat found in animal foods. Diets high in saturated fat and cholesterol may increase the risk of heart disease.

Protein

Protein is needed for growth, maintenance, and repair of body structures, and for the synthesis of regulatory molecules. It can also be broken down to produce energy. Protein is made of folded chains of **amino acids**. The right amounts and types of amino acids must be consumed in the diet to meet the body's protein needs. Animal foods such as meat, poultry, fish, eggs, and dairy products generally supply a combination of amino acids that meets human needs better than plant proteins. However, a vegetarian diet containing only plant foods such as grains, nuts, seeds, vegetables, and legumes can also meet protein needs.

Water

Water is an essential nutrient that makes up about 60% of the adult human body. It provides no energy but is needed in the body to transport nutrients, oxygen, waste products, and other important substances. It also is needed for many chemical reactions, for body structure and protection, and to regulate body temperature. Water is found in beverages as well as in solid foods.

Vitamins

Vitamins are small **organic** molecules needed to regulate metabolic processes. They are found in almost all of the foods we eat, but no one food is a good source of all of them. Some vitamins are soluble in water and others in fat, a property that affects how they are absorbed into and transported throughout the body. Vitamins do not provide energy but many are needed to regulate the chemical reactions that produce usable energy in the body. Some vitamins are **antioxidants**, which protect the body from reactive oxygen compounds like **free radicals**. Others have roles in tissue growth and development, bone health, and blood clotting.

Minerals

Minerals are single **elements**. Some are needed in the diet in significant amounts whereas the requirements for others are extremely small. Like vitamins, minerals provide no energy but perform a number of very diverse functions. Some are needed to regulate chemical reactions, some participate in reactions that protect cells from oxidative reactions, and others have roles in bone formation and maintenance, oxygen transport, or immune function.

HOW MUCH OF EACH NUTRIENT DO YOU NEED?

To stay healthy, adequate amounts of energy and each of the essential nutrients must be consumed in the diet. The amount of each that you need depends on your age, size, sex, genetic makeup, lifestyle, and health status. General guidelines for the amounts of nutrients needed are made by the **Dietary Reference Intakes (DRIs)**. The DRIs were developed by teams of American and Canadian scientists who were asked to review all of the current research and develop recommendations for the amounts of energy, nutrients, and other substances that will best meet needs and maintain health.[1] These recommendations are general guidelines for the amounts of nutrients that should be consumed on an average daily basis in order to promote health, prevent deficiencies, and reduce the incidence of chronic disease. The exact amount of any nutrient that a person needs depends on his or her individual circumstances.

The DRIs

The DRIs include recommendations for amounts of energy, nutrients, and other food components for different groups of people based on age, gender, and, when appropriate, pregnancy and lactation.

The recommendations for energy intakes are expressed as **Estimated Energy Requirements (EERs)**. These can be used to estimate an individual's energy needs (see Appendix A). The recommendations for nutrient intakes include four different types of values. The **Estimated Average Requirement (EAR)** is the amount of a nutrient that is estimated to meet the average needs of the population. It is not used to assess individual intake but is designed for planning and evaluating the adequacy of the nutrient intake of population groups. The **Recommended Dietary Allowances (RDAs)** and **Adequate Intakes (AIs)** are values that are calculated to meet the needs of nearly all healthy people in each gender and life-stage group. These can be used to plan and assess individuals' diets. The fourth set of DRI values is the **Tolerable Upper Intake Levels (ULs)**. These are the maximum levels of intake that are unlikely to pose a risk of adverse health effects. ULs can be used as a guide to limit intake and evaluate the possibility of over-consumption. When your diet provides the RDA or AI for each nutrient and does not exceed the UL for any, your risk of a nutrient deficiency or toxicity is low.

What Happens if You Get Too Little or Too Much?

Consuming either too much or too little of one or more nutrients or energy can cause **malnutrition**. Typically, we think of malnutrition as a deficiency of energy or nutrients. This may occur due to a deficient intake, increased requirements, or an inability to absorb or use nutrients. The effects of malnutrition reflect the function of the nutrient in the body. They may appear rapidly or may take months or years to appear. For example, vitamin D is needed for strong bones. A deficiency causes the leg bones of children to bow outward because they are too weak to support the body weight. Vitamin A is needed for healthy eyes and a deficiency can result in blindness. For many nutrient deficiencies, supplying the deficient nutrient can quickly reverse the symptoms.

Overnutrition, an excess of energy or nutrients, is also a form of malnutrition. An excess of energy causes obesity. It increases the risk of developing diseases such as diabetes and heart disease. Excesses of vitamins and minerals rarely occur from eating food but are most often seen with overuse of dietary supplements. For example, consuming too much vitamin B_6 can cause nerve damage and excess iron intake can cause liver failure.

TOOLS FOR CHOOSING A HEALTHY DIET

Knowing what nutrients your body needs to stay healthy is the first step in choosing a healthy diet, but knowing how many milligrams of niacin, micrograms of vitamin B_{12}, grams of fiber, and what percent of calories from carbohydrate you need does not help you decide what to pack for lunch. Therefore, a variety of tools has been developed to help consumers plan healthy diets. Three of these, Food Labels, the Food Guide Pyramid, and the Dietary Guidelines for Americans, are discussed below. Using each of these tools can help individuals choose the appropriate diets to meet their needs.

Understanding Food Labels

Food labels are a tool designed to help consumers make healthy food choices. They provide information about the nutrient composition of individual foods and how they fit into the recommendations for a healthy diet.

Almost all packaged foods must carry a standard nutrition label. Exceptions are raw fruits, vegetables, fish, meat, and poultry. For these foods, the nutrition information is often posted on placards in the grocery store or printed in brochures. Food labels must include both an ingredient list and a "Nutrition Facts" panel.

FACT BOX 1.3

What Can You Believe?

Product labels and literature often make fabulous claims about the nutritional benefits of the products. Can you believe everything you read? How can you tell what is fact and what is fantasy?

Generally, the rule is, if it sounds too good to be true, it probably is. The following tips offer some suggestions for evaluating nutritional claims:

- **Think about it.** Does the information presented make sense? If not, disregard it.

- **Consider the source.** Where did the information come from? If it is based on personal opinions, be aware that one person's perception does not make something true.

- **Ponder the purpose.** Is the information helping to sell a product? Is it making a magazine cover or newspaper headline more appealing? If so, the claims may be exaggerated to help the sale.

- **View it skeptically.** If a statement claims to be based on a scientific study, think about who did the study, what their credentials are, and what relationship they have to the product. Do they benefit from the sale of the product?

- **Evaluate the risks.** Be sure the expected benefit of the product is worth the risk associated with using it.

Ingredient List

The ingredient list includes all of the substances added when preparing a food, including food additives, colors, and flavorings. The ingredients are listed in order of their prominence by weight. A label that lists water first indicates that most of the weight of that food is water. You can look at the ingredient list if you are trying to avoid certain foods, such as animal products, or a food to which you have an allergy.

Nutrition Facts

The "Nutrition Facts" portion of a food label (Figure 1.2) lists the serving size of the food followed by the total calories, calories from fat, total fat, saturated fat, cholesterol, sodium, total carbohydrate, dietary fiber, sugars, and protein per serving of the food. The amounts of these nutrients are given by weight and as a percentage of the Daily Value. **Daily Values** are standards developed for food labels. They help consumers see how a food fits into their overall diet. For example, if a food provides 10% of the Daily Value for fiber, then the food provides 10% of the daily recommendation for fiber in a 2,000-calorie diet. The amounts of vitamin A, vitamin C, iron, and calcium are also listed as a percentage of the Daily Value.

In addition to the required nutrition information, food labels often highlight specific characteristics of a product that might be of interest to the consumer, such as foods that are "low in calories" or "high in fiber." The Food and Drug Administration (FDA) has developed definitions for these nutrient content descriptors. Food labels are also permitted to include specific health claims if they are relevant. These are only permitted on labels if the scientific evidence for the claim is reviewed by the FDA and found to be factual.

The Food Guide Pyramid

The Food Guide Pyramid (Figure 1.3) is a visual tool for planning your diet that divides foods into five main food groups based on their nutrient composition. Choosing the recommended number of servings from each group and following the selection tips shown in Table 1.1 will provide a diet that meets nutrient requirements and the recommendations for health promotion and disease prevention. The shape of

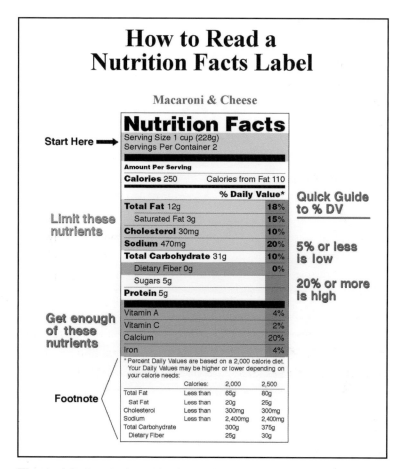

Figure 1.2 Standard nutrition labels like this one appear on all packaged foods. Nutrition labels help people to make informed choices about what they are eating by detailing the amount of each nutrient per serving.

the Pyramid helps emphasize the recommendations for the amounts of food from each of 5 food groups. The wide base of the Pyramid is the Bread, Cereal, Rice, & Pasta Group; choosing between 6 and 11 servings of mostly whole grains forms the foundation of a healthy diet. The next level of the Pyramid includes the Vegetable Group, of which 3 to 5 servings per day are recommended, and the Fruit Group, of which 2 to 4 servings per day are recommended. To meet these recommendations, the 5-a-day health campaign encourages consumers to include

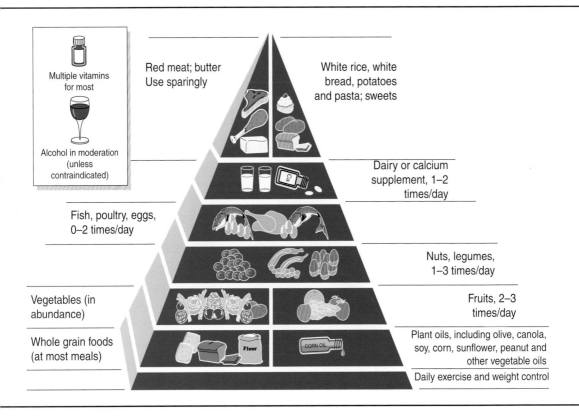

Figure 1.3 The Food Pyramid serves to educate people about how many servings of each food group they should include in their diets. Adapted from the Harvard Food Guide Pyramid.

at least 5 fruits and vegetables in their daily diet. The next level, where the decreasing size of the Pyramid boxes reflects the smaller number of recommended servings, comprises the Milk, Yogurt, & Cheese Group and the Meat, Poultry, Fish, Dry Beans, Eggs, & Nuts Group. Two to 3 servings a day are recommended from each of these groups. The narrow tip of the Pyramid includes a recommendation to use Fats, Oils, & Sweets sparingly in the diet.

The Food Guide Pyramid can be used to plan diets to meet a variety of energy needs. For example, a 100-pound sedentary woman who needs only 1,600 calories per day could meet her needs by choosing 6 servings of breads and cereals, 3 vegetables, 2 fruits, 2 milk servings, and 2 meat servings. In contrast, a 200-pound teenage boy who needs 2,800 calories per day could meet his needs by choosing 11 servings of breads and grains, 5 vegetables, 4 fruits, 3 milk servings, and 3 meat servings. The Pyramid is flexible enough to suit the preferences of people from diverse cultures and lifestyles. For example, a Mexican American might choose tortillas as a grain while a Japanese American might prefer rice; a vegetarian may choose beans from the meat and meat substitute group while someone else might prefer beef.

The Dietary Guidelines

The Dietary Guidelines for Americans is another useful tool that can help you choose a healthy diet. It is a set of recommendations designed to promote health, support active lifestyles, and reduce the risk of chronic disease. It is organized into 3 tiers: the ABCs for Good Health (Figure 1.4).

The first tier, called "Aim for Fitness," includes two guidelines that recommend that we "Aim for a healthy weight" and "Be physically active each day." These recommendations are backed up by specific guidelines for body weight and activity levels.

The "Build a Healthy Base" tier offers four guidelines on choosing a variety of foods and handling these foods safely. It recommends that we let the Food Pyramid guide our food choices; eat a variety of grains, especially whole grains, daily; eat a variety of fruits and vegetables daily; and "Keep food safe to eat."

The last tier, "Choose Sensibly," recommends limiting intakes of certain dietary components. The first guideline, "Choose a diet low in saturated fat and cholesterol and moderate in total fat," reflects the understanding that diets low in saturated fat and cholesterol may reduce the risk of heart disease. The guideline to "Choose beverages and foods that limit your intake of sugars" is based on the fact that the consumption of sugar in the United States has been on the rise and may be increasing the incidence of chronic disease. "Choose and prepare foods with less salt" is based on research that indicates that a diet high in salt increases blood pressure in some individuals. The final guideline emphasizes the dangers of excess alcohol consumption.

Table 1.1 Servings and Selections From the Food Guide Pyramid

FOOD GROUP/SERVING SIZE	NUTRIENTS PROVIDED	SELECTION TIPS
Bread, Cereal, Rice, & Pasta (6 to 11 servings) 1/2 cup cooked cereal, rice, or pasta 1 ounce dry cereal 1 slice bread 1 tortilla 2 cookies 1/2 medium doughnut	B vitamins Fiber Iron Magnesium Zinc Complex carbohydrate	• Choose whole-grain breads, cereals, and grains such as whole wheat or rye, oatmeal, and brown rice. • Use high-fat, high-sugar baked goods such as cakes, cookies, and pastries in moderation. • Limit fats and sugars added as spreads, sauces, or toppings.
Vegetable (3 to 5 servings) 1/2 cup cooked or raw chopped vegetables 1 cup raw leafy vegetables 3/4 cup vegetable juice 10 french fries	Vitamin A Vitamin C Folate Magnesium Iron Fiber	• Eat a variety of vegetables, including dark-green leafy vegetables like spinach and broccoli, deep-yellow vegetables like carrots and sweet potatoes, starchy vegetables such as potatoes and corn, and other vegetables such as green beans and tomatoes. • Cook by steaming or baking. • Avoid frying, and limit high-fat spreads or dressings.
Fruit (2 to 4 servings) 1 medium apple, banana, or orange 1/2 cup chopped, cooked, or canned fruit 3/4 cup fruit juice 1/4 cup dried fruit	Vitamin A Vitamin C Potassium Fiber	• Choose fresh fruit, frozen fruit without sugar, dried fruit, or fruit canned in water or juice. • If canned in heavy syrup, rinse fruit with water before eating. • Eat whole fruits more often than juices; they are higher in fiber. • Regularly eat citrus fruits, melons, or berries rich in vitamin C. • Only 100% fruit juice should be counted as fruit.
Milk, Yogurt, & Cheese (2 to 3 servings) 1 cup milk or yogurt 1-1/2 ounces natural cheese 2 ounces processed cheese 2 cups cottage cheese 1-1/2 cups ice cream 1 cup frozen yogurt	Protein Calcium Riboflavin Vitamin D	• Use low-fat or skim milk for healthy people over 2 years of age. • Choose low-fat and nonfat yogurt, "part skim"and low-fat cheeses, and lower-fat frozen desserts like ice milk and frozen yogurt. • Limit high-fat cheeses and ice cream.

FOOD GROUP/SERVING SIZE	NUTRIENTS PROVIDED	SELECTION TIPS
Meat, Poultry, Fish, Dry Beans, Eggs, & Nuts **(2 to 3 servings)** 2–3 ounces cooked lean meat, fish, or poultry 2–3 eggs 4–6 tablespoons peanut butter 1 to 1-1/2 cups cooked dry beans 2/3 to 1 cup nuts	Protein Niacin Vitamin B_6 Vitamin B_{12} Other B vitamins Iron Zinc	• Select lean meat, poultry without skin, and dry beans often. • Trim fat, and cook by broiling, roasting, grilling, or boiling rather than frying. • Limit egg yolks, which are high in cholesterol, and nuts and seeds, which are high in fat. • Be aware of serving size; 3 ounces of meat is the size of an average hamburger.
Fats, Oils, & Sweets **(use sparingly)** Butter Mayonnaise Salad dressing Cream cheese Sour cream Jam Jelly	Fat-soluble vitamins	• These are high in energy and low in micronutrients. • Substitute low-fat dressings and spreads.

Human Nutrition Information Service. *The Food Guide Pyramid*. Home and Garden Bulletin No. 252. Hyattsville, MD: U.S. Department of Agriculture, 1992, 1996, revised.

CONNECTIONS

Human nutrition is the science that studies the interactions between people and food. Food provides nutrients, which are substances required in the diet for growth, reproduction, and maintenance of the body. There are six classes of nutrients. Carbohydrate includes sugars, starches, and fibers. Sugars and starches provide energy, 4 calories per gram. Fibers provide little energy because they cannot be digested by human enzymes and therefore cannot be absorbed. Lipids are a concentrated source of calories in the diet and in the body, providing 9 calories per gram. They are also needed to synthesize structural and regulatory molecules. Proteins are made from amino acids. In the body, proteins can

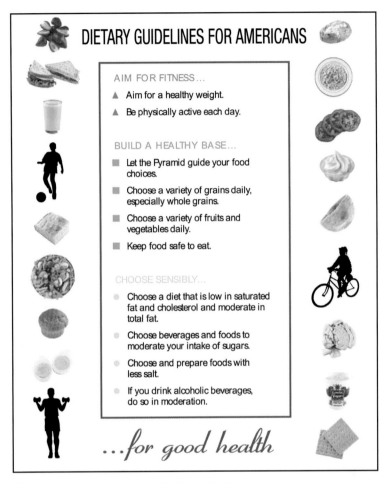

Figure 1.4 The Dietary Guidelines for Americans can help a person choose a healthy and sensible diet. These guidelines suggest that people get enough exercise; choose a variety of different, healthy foods; and limit intake of certain food components such as sugar, salt, and cholesterol.

provide energy but are more important for their structural and regulatory roles. Water is the most abundant nutrient in the body. Water intake must equal output to maintain balance. Vitamins and minerals are needed in the diet in small amounts. They both have regulatory roles and some minerals also provide structure. Consuming too much or too little energy or nutrients results in malnutrition. The Dietary Reference Intakes (DRIs) recommend amounts of energy and nutrients needed to promote health, prevent deficiencies, and reduce the incidence of chronic disease. The Daily Values on Food Labels, the Food Guide Pyramid, and the Dietary Guidelines for Americans present recommendations for choosing foods that will provide these nutrients.

FACT BOX 1.4

How Healthy Is the American Diet?

A healthy diet should be based on whole grains, vegetables, and fruits, with smaller amounts of dairy products and high-protein foods and limited amounts of fats and sweets. In general, the American diet does not meet these recommendations. The Dietary Guidelines and the Food Guide Pyramid recommend that we choose whole rather than refined grains, but the average American consumes only one serving of whole grains per day. The Food Guide Pyramid recommends 2–4 servings of fruit, but the average person eats only 1-2/3 servings each day and 48% of Americans do not even consume one piece of fruit daily. We also fall short of the 2–3 servings of dairy products recommended. Americans on average eat only 1-1/2 dairy servings daily, and only 12% of teenage girls and 14% of women consume the recommended amounts.[a] In addition to missing out on the benefits of whole grain and fruit, we eat too much added sugar. The average American consumes about 64 pounds of sugar a year or about 20 teaspoons a day of added sugar, mostly from soft drinks. Americans drink over 13 billion gallons of carbonated beverages every year.[b] The typical American diet, along with a lack of physical activity, contributes to the development of chronic diseases, such as diabetes, obesity, heart disease, and cancer, which are the major causes of illness and death in the population of the United States. One estimate suggests that 14% of all premature deaths in the United States can be attributed to diet and a sedentary lifestyle. Recommendations for reducing disease risk focus on increasing activity patterns and choosing a diet that meets recommendations.

a Cleveland, E., Cook, J.E., Wilson, J.W., et al. Pyramid Servings Data from the 1994 CSFII data ARS Food Survey Research. Available online at *www.barc.usda.gov/bhnrc/foodsurveys/home.html*. Accessed May 30, 2003.

b "Pouring Rights: Marketing Empty Calories." Public Health Reports 2000. Vol. 115. Oxford University Press, 2000, pp. 308–319.

2

Carbohydrates

High-carbohydrate foods are the basis of diets around the world. Rice is the staple in the Asian diet, pasta in Italian cuisine, and corn or wheat tortillas in the diets of South Americans. Whether the diet is that of a farmer in China or an aristocrat in England, the greatest proportion of calories generally comes from carbohydrates. This has been true for centuries. Nonetheless, diets high in carbohydrates have been blamed for everything from obesity to hyperactivity. The reason for this is related to the types and sources of carbohydrates we include in our diet.

WHAT IS A CARBOHYDRATE?

The basic unit of carbohydrate is a single **sugar** molecule. All other carbohydrates are made up of two or more sugars linked together. Single sugars are called **monosaccharides**. The three most common monosaccharides in the diet are **glucose**, **fructose**, and **galactose**. Each contains 6 carbon, 12 hydrogen, and 6 oxygen atoms, but the arrangement is different for each sugar. Glucose is the form of sugar that travels in our bloodstream; it is often called blood sugar. Fructose is the form of sugar found in fruit; it is called fruit sugar. Galactose is a component of the sugar that is found in milk.

When two sugar molecules are linked together, they form a **disaccharide**. The most common disaccharides in the diet are **lactose**, **maltose**, and **sucrose**. Lactose, or milk sugar, is the only sugar found naturally in animal foods; it is made up of glucose linked to galactose. Maltose consists of two molecules of glucose. Sucrose is what we know as common white table sugar; it is formed by linking glucose to fructose.

The mono- and disaccharides together are known as **simple carbohydrates**. When many sugar molecules are linked together, they form a **polysaccharide** (*poly* means "many") (Figure 2.1). Polysaccharides are also called **complex carbohydrates**. They are found in plant foods and include starches and fibers. We consume starch in vegetables like potatoes, beans, and corn, where it is an energy storage molecule for the plant. Fibers, such as those in the skins of fruits, are complex carbohydrates that cannot be digested by human enzymes. The role of fiber in human nutrition will be discussed in the following chapter. **Glycogen**, sometimes called animal starch, is a polysaccharide found in humans and other animals. It is made of glucose molecules linked together in highly branched chains. This branched structure allows it to be broken down quickly, to release glucose into the blood when it is needed. We do not consume much glycogen in our diets because the molecule breaks down after the animal dies.

CARBOHYDRATE IN OUR DIETS

Carbohydrate makes up more than 50% of the energy in a typical American's diet. Some of this is simple carbohydrate and some is complex. Some is unrefined, meaning it is consumed from its natural source, and some is refined and added to foods. Recommendations for a healthy diet suggest that we eat more carbohydrates from their natural sources and limit our consumption of refined carbohydrate and added sugars.

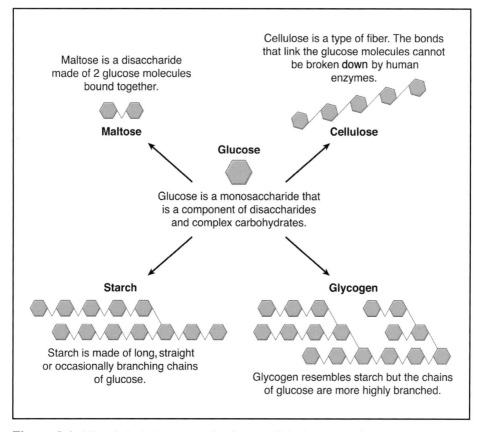

Figure 2.1 All carbohydrates are made of sugars linked together. Some common carbohydrates and their composition are illustrated here.

Sweet and Simple Sugars

Sugars are sweet. We eat them in both natural and refined forms in our diets. Natural sources include the fructose in fruit and the lactose in dairy products. Refined sources include table sugar, high-fructose corn syrup, corn syrup, maltose, and honey (honey is refined by bees) that are added to foods in processing or at the table. Although refined sugars are chemically no different from natural ones, they are considered **empty calories** because they provide energy but contain few other nutrients. Because sucrose is the only sweetener that can be called "sugar" in the ingredient list on food labels in the United States, you need to know the names of other added sweeteners in order to see if sugars have been added to a food.

Is It Better to Be Complex?

In North America, we consume most of our complex carbohydrate as grains such as wheat, rice, and corn. These contain both starches and

---

FACT BOX 2.1

Glycogen—Topping off the Tank

Glycogen stored in muscles provides fuel for exercise. The more glycogen you have and the more slowly you use it, the longer you can exercise before you run out of gas. To top off the tank before serious competition, endurance athletes often follow a regimen of glycogen supercompensation, also known as carbohydrate loading. The goal is to empty muscle glycogen stores by exercising and then fill them up by cutting back on exercise and eating a very high-carbohydrate diet for a few days before competition. The process takes a total of six days. For the first three days, a diet containing about 50% carbohydrates is consumed. This is then increased to 70% carbohydrates for the last three days. The workout on the first day should last about 90 minutes and then workouts should be gradually tapered down; day six, the day before competition, is a rest day. This regimen will increase the amount of muscle glycogen from about 1.7 grams of glycogen per 100 grams of muscle to 4 to 5 grams per 100 grams.[a]

Glycogen supercompensation is beneficial to endurance athletes, but it may not be the best thing for you. If your athletic activities last less than an hour, this regimen will provide no benefit and even has some disadvantages. For every gram of glycogen in the muscle, almost 3 grams of water are also deposited. The water with the extra glycogen will cause you to gain 2 to 7 pounds and may cause some muscle stiffness. As glycogen is used, the water is released. Although this can be an advantage when exercising in hot weather, carrying the extra weight may cancel out any potential benefits from increased energy stores, especially for short-duration events.

a McArdle, W.D., Katch, F.I., and Katch, V.L. *Exercise Physiology: Energy, Nutrition and Human Performance*, 5th ed. Baltimore, MD: Lippincott Williams & Wilkins, 2001, p. 578.

fiber, but the amount of each varies depending on the food and how it has been processed. A plate of pasta, a slice of bread, and a bowl of rice are all good sources of starch, but unless they are whole-wheat pasta, whole-wheat bread, and brown rice, they are not good sources of fiber. This is because the fiber has been removed during the refining of the grain. A kernel of grain has outer layers called the **bran**, which are

---

FACT BOX 2.2

The Case of the Strawberry Yogurt

How much sugar is in a container of strawberry yogurt? It doesn't take a detective to find the answer. The number of grams of sugars in a serving is listed on the Nutrition Facts label; a cup of strawberry yogurt has 37 grams. But this number doesn't tell you whether the sugar came from the milk and strawberries used to make the yogurt, or if it was added to sweeten the final product. The 37 grams listed on the label includes the fructose found naturally in strawberries, the lactose found naturally in milk, and any sugars added in processing. There is no way to know for sure from the Nutrition Facts label how much of the total is made up of added sugars. Sometimes a label will say "no added sugar" or "without added sugar"—this tells you that no sugars were added in processing. Sometimes the ingredient list provides some information about the sweeteners added to a food. Only added sugars are listed here. The weights of ingredients are not given, but ingredients are listed in order of prominence by weight, so the closer an ingredient is to the top of the list, the more of it there is in the food. In the strawberry yogurt, sugar is the second ingredient. This means that sucrose, the only sugar that can rightly be called "sugar" in the ingredients list, is present in the second greatest amount by weight of all the ingredients used in making the yogurt. There may be other sugars used, but to find them, you need to increase your sugar vocabulary. High-fructose corn syrups, invert sugar, dextrose, lactose, and honey are just a few. In the strawberry yogurt, sugar is the second ingredient and high-fructose corn syrup is the fourth ingredient. The amount of added sugar is the sum of these two sources of sugar. If you are looking for a product without added sugars, check the ingredients list to be sure you know what you are getting.

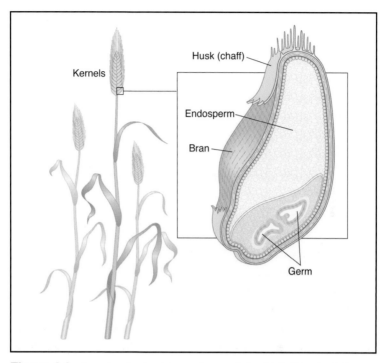

Figure 2.2 A grain of wheat is made up of the high-fiber bran layers, the starchy endosperm, and the oil-rich germ.

high in fiber; an oil-rich structure called the **germ** located at the base of the kernel; and a large central portion called the **endosperm**, which contains most of the starch (Figure 2.2). Whole-grain products are made from the entire kernel, including the bran, germ, and endosperm. Refined grains, such as white flour, are made by removing the bran and the germ to produce a more uniform product. Removing the bran and germ, however, also removes fiber, vitamins, and minerals.

Legumes, such as kidney beans and black-eyed peas, and starchy vegetables, such as corn and potatoes, are also good sources of complex carbohydrate. Legumes are high in fiber but potatoes and other tubers are mostly starch. Other vegetables, such as tomatoes, broccoli, and green beans, contain less starch and more fiber. Starches are added as thickeners to foods such as sauces, puddings, and gravies because starch granules swell when heated with water.

HOW IS CARBOHYDRATE DIGESTED?

To be absorbed into the body, all carbohydrate, whether simple or complex, must be broken down into monosaccharides. This break-down, or digestion, occurs with the help of enzymes throughout the digestive tract. The digestion of starch begins in the mouth, where the enzyme **salivary amylase** breaks it into shorter polysaccharides. Starch digestion continues in the small intestine, where the action of pancreatic amylases breaks polysaccharides into maltose. Enzymes attached to the lining of the small intestine then complete the digestion of maltose and also break sucrose and lactose into monosaccharides. The monosaccharides glucose, galactose, and fructose are then absorbed into the blood and transported to the liver.

If carbohydrate in the small intestine is not completely digested to monosaccharides, it cannot be absorbed and passes into the large intestine. Here, some of the carbohydrate is digested by bacteria. This produces acids, gas, and other by-products, which may cause abdominal discomfort and flatulence. The reason beans cause flatulence is that they contain short polysaccharides called **oligosaccharides** that cannot be completely digested by human enzymes and, thus, pass into the large intestine. This is also the reason why people who have **lactose intolerance** are not able to consume milk or other dairy products without experiencing symptoms such as abdominal distension, flatulence, cramping, and diarrhea. In lactose intolerant individuals, the level of intestinal lactase, the enzyme that breaks down lactose, is reduced. Lactase is normally produced by all humans at birth and the activity of the enzyme decreases with age; in many individuals, it declines so much that lactose cannot be completely digested. It is estimated that about 25% of adults in the United States are lactose intolerant; the incidence is about 80% for African Americans and 90% for Asian Americans. Most individuals who are lactose intolerant can consume small amounts of lactose without experiencing symptoms. Yogurt and cheese are more easily tolerated than milk because some of the lactose in these products is digested or lost in processing. Lactase tablets, which digest the lactose before it passes into the large intestine, are also available.

WHAT DO CARBOHYDRATES DO?

Carbohydrate serves a number of functions in the body. The sugar galactose is needed in nervous tissue and to make lactose in breast milk; the monosaccharides deoxyribose and ribose are needed to make DNA and RNA, which contain the genetic information for the synthesis of proteins; and short polysaccharides are important signaling molecules found on the surface of cells. The main role of carbohydrate, though, particularly glucose, is as an energy source, providing about 4 calories per gram. Certain body cells, including brain cells and red blood cells, rely almost exclusively on glucose for energy.

Because of the key role glucose plays in providing energy to body cells, the level of glucose in the blood, and therefore the amount available to the cells, is carefully regulated. Normal blood glucose levels are about 60 to 100 mg per 100 ml of blood. This level is regulated primarily by the hormones **insulin** and **glucagon**. A rise in blood glucose, which occurs after eating carbohydrate, triggers the pancreas to secrete insulin. Insulin promotes the uptake of glucose by body cells, where it can be used for energy production or stored as glycogen for later use. This removes glucose from the blood, decreasing blood glucose levels to the normal range. The disease **diabetes** occurs when these regulatory mechanisms fail, allowing blood glucose levels to remain high. The high glucose concentration can damage the eyes, the kidneys, and the circulatory and nervous systems.

When blood glucose drops too low, glucagon causes liver glycogen to break down, releasing glucose into the blood. Glucagon also stimulates liver and kidney cells to synthesize new glucose molecules by a process known as **gluconeogenesis**. Gluconeogenesis is important for meeting the body's need for glucose, but the 3-carbon molecules it uses to synthesize glucose come primarily from amino acids found in body proteins. It therefore uses up protein that could be used for other essential functions. When carbohydrate intake is adequate in the diet, protein is not needed to synthesize glucose. Therefore, carbohydrate is said to spare protein. Glucose cannot be synthesized from fatty acids because they break down to form 2-carbon rather than 3-carbon molecules.

CARBOHYDRATE METABOLISM:
USING CARBOHYDRATE FOR ENERGY

Once glucose reaches the cells, it is broken down via a series of reactions called **cellular respiration** to produce carbon dioxide, water, and energy in the form of ATP. Cellular respiration involves four stages (Figure 2.3). The first stage is called **glycolysis**. In glycolysis, the 6-carbon sugar glucose is broken into two 3-carbon **pyruvate** molecules, and 2 molecules of ATP are produced. This stage is referred to as **anaerobic** glycolysis or anaerobic metabolism because it can proceed whether or not oxygen is available in the cells. It produces ATP from glucose rapidly but inefficiently. What happens to the pyruvate molecules next depends on whether or not oxygen is available at the cells. When oxygen is unavailable, the pyruvate produced by anaerobic metabolism is converted to **lactic acid**. During intense exercise, lactic acid can accumulate in the muscles, causing muscle cramping and fatigue. When oxygen is available, cellular respiration can proceed.

The second stage of cellular respiration involves the conversion of pyruvate to **acetyl CoA**. Acetyl CoA then enters the third stage, the citric acid cycle, where it combines with a 4-carbon molecule called oxaloacetate. In the citric acid cycle, single carbons are removed as carbon dioxide until oxaloacetate is reformed. During these first three stages of cellular respiration, electrons are released. In the presence of oxygen, these are passed to the final stage of cellular respiration, the **electron transport chain**. The electron transport chain accepts the

---

FACT BOX 2.3

Diabetes on the Rise

The incidence of diabetes in the United States is increasing. Most of this increase is in type 2 diabetes, the form of the disease that is thought to be related to lifestyle. Type 2 diabetes used to be considered a problem only in adults age 40 and older, but it is now increasing drastically in children and young adults. The reason for this is believed to be related to the increase in obesity among children and teens.

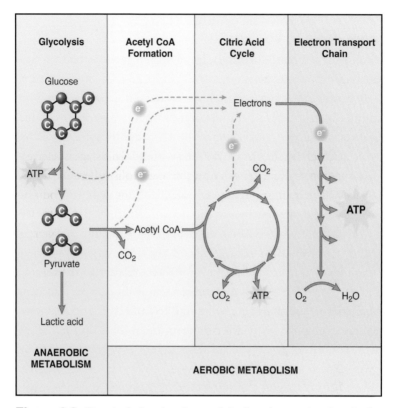

Figure 2.3 Glycolysis breaks glucose into 3-carbon molecules. In the presence of oxygen, these are converted to acetyl CoA, which enters the citric acid cycle. High-energy electrons are released and transferred to the electron transport chain, where their energy is trapped to make ATP.

electrons and passes them down a chain of molecules until they are finally combined with oxygen to form water. As the electrons are passed along, their energy is trapped and used to make ATP. Because oxygen is required for the last three stages of cellular respiration to proceed, they are referred to as **aerobic metabolism**. Aerobic metabolism, which completely breaks down glucose to form carbon dioxide, water, and ATP, produces about 38 molecules of ATP per molecule of glucose. In contrast, when no oxygen is available and glucose is broken down by anaerobic metabolism, only 2 molecules of ATP are produced from each glucose molecule.

SO IS A DIET HIGH IN CARBOHYDRATE GOOD OR BAD FOR YOU?

A diet high in carbohydrate can be either good or bad for you depending on the types of carbohydrate that are consumed as well as the other components of the diet. In general, diets high in unrefined sources of carbohydrate such as whole grains, fruits, and vegetables are considered healthy because they are associated with a lower incidence of a variety of bowel disorders, heart disease, diabetes, and certain cancers, whereas diets high in added sugars and refined grains are generally considered unhealthy. This is because they are low in nutrient density. **Nutrient density** refers to the amounts of essential nutrients relative to the amount of energy. Foods like donuts, cakes, and cookies are low in nutrient density because they contain few nutrients relative to the calories they provide. Diets high in refined carbohydrate have also been blamed for tooth decay, hyperactivity, obesity, and diabetes. Research supports a role for carbohydrate in some, but not all of, these conditions.

Does Sugar Cause Cavities?

The most common health problem associated with a diet high in simple carbohydrate is dental caries or cavities. Dental caries are formed when bacteria that live in the mouth metabolize sugar from the diet and produce acid. The acid can then dissolve the enamel and underlying structure of the teeth. Simple carbohydrates, particularly sucrose, cause cavities because they are the favorite food source for these bacteria, but starch can also be metabolized into cavity-forming acid. Preventing cavities requires proper dental hygiene even if the diet is low in sugar.

Does Sugar Make You Hyper?

Sugar consumption has also been suggested as a cause of hyperactivity in children. However, research on sugar intake and behavior has failed to support the connection between sugar and hyperactivity.[2] Other factors, including caffeine consumption, lack of either physical activity or sleep, and overstimulation, are likely to play a role.

Do Sweets and Starchy Foods Make You Fat?

Carbohydrates have been accused of contributing to weight gain. Based just on calories, this seems unlikely. Carbohydrates provide only 4 calories per gram compared to 9 calories per gram for fat. However, it has been suggested that because eating carbohydrate stimulates the release of insulin and insulin removes glucose from the blood and promotes energy storage, diets high in carbohydrate may increase both hunger and the storage of body fat. Even if this occurs, the bottom line on weight gain is that it is caused by consuming more calories than are expended. As long as calorie intake does not exceed calorie needs, weight will not increase. Unrefined carbohydrates, which are high in fiber, may actually promote weight loss because the fiber they provide makes you feel full after fewer calories are consumed.

Do Refined Carbohydrates Cause Diabetes?

Evidence is accumulating that long-term consumption of a diet high in refined starches and added sugars may increase the risk of developing diabetes. When refined starches and added sugars are consumed, blood glucose and, subsequently, insulin levels in the blood rise more sharply than when unrefined carbohydrates are eaten. This increased demand for insulin has been suggested as a factor for increasing the risk of developing diabetes. In fact, diabetes is less common in populations that consume diets high in unrefined grains (Figure 2.4).[3]

HOW MUCH OF WHAT KIND OF CARBOHYDRATE DO YOU NEED?

In order to keep glucose available to cells, a minimal amount of carbohydrate is needed. To meet this need, the DRIs recommend at least 150 grams of carbohydrate per day. However, in order to meet energy needs without consuming too much fat or protein, the DRIs suggest that a healthy diet provide between 45% and 65% of calories from carbohydrate.[4] This is equivalent to 225 to 325 grams of carbohydrate for someone who eats 2,000 calories a day.

The typical American diet contains about 52% of calories as carbohydrate. This amount is within the recommended range of 45% to 65%; however, the types of carbohydrate that Americans consume

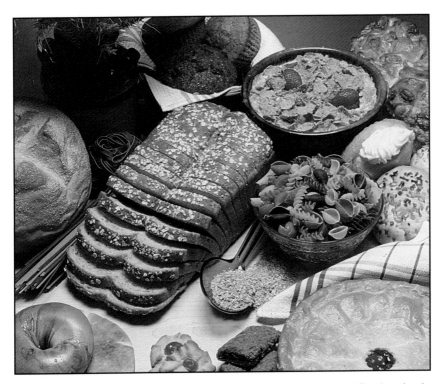

Figure 2.4 Your long-term health may be improved by replacing refined grains in your diet, such as the cookies and pie in this photo, with less refined grain products, such as the whole-grain muffins and whole-wheat bread.

do not meet public health guidelines. Recommendations suggest that we limit added sugar consumption to less than 10% of calories, but it is estimated that 16% to 20% of our calories come from added sugars in foods such as soft drinks, candy, and bakery products.[4] It is recommended that we consume whole grains such as whole-wheat bread, brown rice, and oatmeal rather than refined grain products like white bread, white rice, and sugared breakfast cereals, but the average American consumes only one serving of whole grains per day.

CONNECTIONS

Carbohydrate includes sugars, starches, and fibers; sugars and starches provide energy, at a rate of 4 calories per gram. Sugars are called simple carbohydrates and include single sugars called monosaccharides and double sugars called disaccharides. Sugars in our diet include those naturally found in fruits and milk and those added to foods in processing and at the table. Starches are found in grains, legumes, and starchy vegetables. They are made of chains of glucose molecules and are broken down to glucose in the digestive tract to be absorbed. In the body, glucose is metabolized to produce ATP, the energy source required by cells. To ensure a constant supply of glucose to body cells, blood glucose levels are regulated by the hormones insulin and glucagon. Recommendations suggest people should have a minimum carbohydrate intake of 150 grams per day, but a more realistic goal is 45% to 65% of calories from carbohydrate. This should come primarily from whole grains, fruits, vegetables, and milk with limited amounts of added sugars. A diet that meets these recommendations may reduce the risk of diabetes and dental caries.

FACT BOX 2.4

Artificial Sweeteners: Satisfying Your Sweet Tooth

If you love sweets but don't like the calories they add to your diet, you might try artificial sweeteners. A 12-ounce sugar-sweetened soft drink has about 150 calories. A soft drink made with artificial sweeteners has almost none. There are four artificial sweeteners used in foods sold in the United States: saccharine, aspartame, Acelsufame K, and sucralose. They can sweeten food without adding many calories and they are generally safe for healthy people. If you replace some foods that are high in added sugars with artificially sweetened products, you can cut down on calories and decrease your sugar intake, but you will not necessarily make your diet healthier. Whether the soft drink is sweetened with sugar or artificial sweeteners, it provides no other nutrients to the diet. A healthy diet is based on foods such as whole grains, vegetables, and fruits that provide many nutrients relative to the calories they contain.

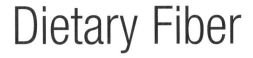

3

Dietary Fiber

Eat your roughage—that's what your grandparents told you.
What they called roughage is what we call fiber. Fiber is plant matter
that cannot be digested by human enzymes. We consume it in whole
grains, legumes, fruits, and vegetables. Because we cannot digest it,
fiber moves through the digestive system and is excreted in the feces.
However, even though it is not absorbed, it is important to our health.

TYPES OF FIBER IN THE DIET

Fiber includes a number of chemical substances that have different
physical properties and physiological effects in the body. Most fibers
are indigestible carbohydrate, but lignin, which is chemically
not a carbohydrate, is also classified as fiber. This is because of the
way it behaves in the digestive tract. Fibers have traditionally been
categorized based on their solubility in water.

Insoluble fibers are those that do not dissolve in water. They are
derived primarily from the structural parts of plants, such as the
cell walls. Chemically, they include lignin and cellulose and some

Table 3.1 Dietary Sources of Soluble and Insoluble Fiber

FOOD/SERVING	TOTAL FIBER (g)	INSOLUBLE FIBER (g)	SOLUBLE FIBER (g)	ENERGY (Cal)
Wheat bran flakes, 1 cup	6.15	5.52	0.63	126
Broccoli, 1 cup	2.80	1.40	1.40	28
Celery, 1 stalk	0.29	0.19	0.10	3
Oatmeal, 1 cup	4.00	2.15	1.85	145
Apple, 1 medium	3.73	2.76	0.97	81
Carrot, 1 medium	1.84	0.92	0.92	26
Plum, 1 medium	0.99	0.46	0.53	36
Kidney beans, 1/2 cup	5.72	2.86	2.86	113
Green peas, 1/2 cup	4.40	3.12	1.28	62
Metamucil, 1 Tbsp	5.10	1.05	4.05	21

hemicelluloses. Dietary sources of insoluble fiber include wheat bran and rye bran, and vegetables such as broccoli.

Soluble fibers form viscous solutions when placed in water. They are found in and around plant cells and include pectins, gums, and some hemicelluloses. Food sources of soluble fibers include oats, apples, beans, and seaweed. Soluble fibers are often added to foods in processing. Pectin is used to thicken jams and jellies. Gums, such as gum arabic, gum karaya, guar gum, locust bean gum, xanthan gum, and gum tragacanth, come from shrubs, trees, and seed pods. Agar, carrageenan, and alginates come from seaweed, and are used as thickeners and stabilizers in foods like salad dressing and ice cream. Pectins and gums are also used in reduced-fat products because they mimic the texture of fat. Most foods of plant origin contain mixtures of soluble and insoluble fibers (Table 3.1 and Figure 3.1).

WHAT HAPPENS TO FIBER IN THE DIGESTIVE TRACT?

Because fiber cannot be digested, it travels through the gastrointestinal (GI) tract and is excreted in the feces. Soluble and insoluble

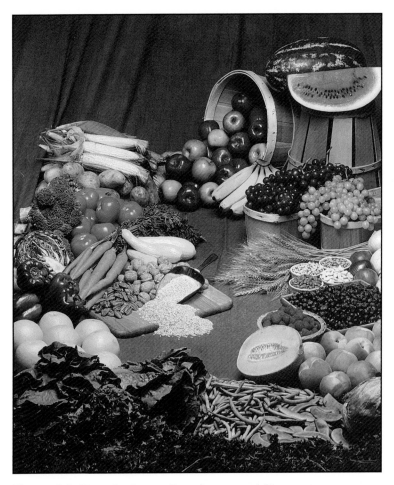

Figure 3.1 These foods are all good sources of fiber.

fibers behave somewhat differently in the gastrointestinal tract. Soluble fibers absorb water and form viscous solutions that slow the rate at which nutrients are absorbed. In the colon, bacteria can digest soluble fibers producing gas and fatty acids, small quantities of which can be absorbed and affect other functions in the body. Insoluble fibers do not attract water and are not broken down by bacteria but they do increase the amount of material in the intestine. When consumed together, the increased bulk of insoluble fiber and the water associated with soluble fiber increase the volume of material in the intestine. This allows for easier passage of the stool and speeds transit time, which is the time it takes food and fecal matter to move through the gastrointestinal tract. It also strengthens the muscles of the colon by stimulating the rhythmic muscle contractions called **peristalsis** that propel food through the digestive tract.

HOW DOES FIBER AFFECT YOUR HEALTH?

A diet high in fiber has beneficial effects on the health of the gastrointestinal tract and can relieve or prevent some chronic health problems. When a high-fiber diet is consumed, the feces are larger and softer and the amount of pressure needed for defecation is reduced. This helps reduce the incidence of constipation, defined as infrequent stools that are dry and difficult to pass. It also prevents hemorrhoids, which are swellings of the veins in the rectal or anal area. The reduced pressure in the large intestine also reduces the risk of **diverticulosis** (Figure 3.2), a condition in which outpouchings form in the intestinal wall. If fecal matter accumulates in these out-pouchings, it can cause irritation, pain, inflammation, and infection, a condition known as diverticulitis.

FACT BOX 3.1

Fiber Gets Things Moving

A high-fiber diet increases the volume of fecal matter and the rate at which it moves through the gastrointestinal tract. When African villagers who ate a high-fiber diet were compared with British people who ate a low-fiber diet, the differing effects of these diets were striking. It took an average of only about 35 hours for material to pass through the digestive tracts of the African villagers, but it took almost 70 hours for material to move through the digestive tracts of the British subjects. Dramatic differences were also seen in stool weight. Those eating the high-fiber diets had an average daily stool weight of about 480 grams in contrast to only about 110 grams for the low-fiber diet. The greater fecal volume and shorter transit time is thought to reduce the exposure of intestinal cells to potentially harmful materials.

From Burkitt, D.P., Walker, A.R.P., and Painter, N.S. "Dietary fiber and disease." *Journal of the American Medical Association* 229: 1068–1074, 1974.

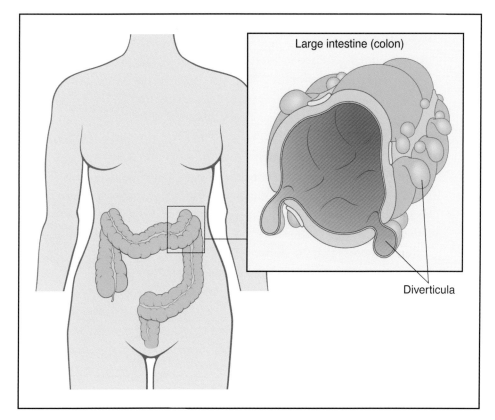

Figure 3.2 A diagram of diverticula in the colon is shown here. The risk of developing diverticulosis is increased by consuming a low-fiber diet.

Fiber Can Reduce Blood Cholesterol

A diet high in fiber can help reduce blood cholesterol levels and thereby reduce the risk of heart disease. Soluble fibers such as those in legumes, rice and oat bran, gums, pectin, and psyllium (a grain used in over-the-counter bulk-forming laxatives such as Metamucil) bind cholesterol and **bile acids** in the digestive tract, preventing their absorption. Bile acids, which are made from cholesterol, are secreted into the GI tract, where they are needed for the absorption of dietary fat. Normally, the bile acids are absorbed with the fat and reused. However, when soluble fiber is present, it binds to the bile acids and cholesterol, causing them to be excreted in the feces rather than being absorbed. The liver must then use cholesterol from the blood to synthesize new bile acids, thereby reducing blood cholesterol levels. Another reason soluble fiber may help reduce blood cholesterol is because the short chain fatty acids produced by the microbial digestion of fiber may inhibit cholesterol synthesis.[1,5]

Fiber and Diabetes

A high-fiber diet is beneficial for the prevention and management of diabetes. The added bulk and thick solutions formed by fiber in the intestine slows the absorption of nutrients, including glucose. Therefore, blood glucose levels will rise more slowly when a carbohydrate-containing meal is high in fiber. This decreases the amount of insulin needed to keep glucose in the normal range. This is beneficial for managing blood glucose in individuals with diabetes and over the long term is believed to reduce the risk of developing diabetes. This is supported by studies that have found that diets high in fiber are associated with a lower incidence of diabetes.

Fiber and Colon Cancer

Adequate dietary fiber may protect against colon cancer. Epidemiological studies have shown that colon cancer incidence is lower in populations that consume high-fiber diets. This may occur because fiber dilutes the intestinal contents and speeds the rate at which material moves through the intestines. Together, these effects decrease the amount of time that the cells lining the intestine are in contact with potentially cancer-causing substances present in the intestinal contents. The presence of fiber in the intestine may also change the type of bacteria that grow there and the substances produced by the bacteria as they break down material in the colon. These substances may directly affect cells in the colon. Some of the effect of a high-fiber diet on colon cancer may also be due to substances other than fiber that are present in high-fiber foods.

Problems With High Fiber

A high-fiber diet can cause problems if fluid intake is not sufficient or if fiber is increased too rapidly. High-fiber diets also have the potential to affect vitamin and mineral status and calorie intake.

When fiber is consumed without enough fluid, it can cause constipation. Fiber increases water needs because it holds fluid in the gastrointestinal tract. The more fiber there is in the diet, the more water is needed to keep the stool soft. When too little fluid is consumed, the stool becomes hard and difficult to eliminate. In severe cases when fiber intake is excessive and fluid intake is low, intestinal blockage can occur. To avoid these problems, the fiber and fluid content of the diet should be increased gradually. Even when there is plenty of fluid, a sudden increase in the fiber content of the diet can cause abdominal discomfort, gas, and diarrhea due to the bacterial breakdown of fiber.

In some individuals, a diet high in fiber can increase the risk of vitamin and mineral deficiencies. This occurs for two reasons. First, the increase in the volume of intestinal contents that occurs with a high-fiber diet may prevent enzymes from coming in contact with food. If a food cannot be broken down, the vitamins and minerals from that food cannot be absorbed. Second, fiber may bind some micronutrients, preventing their absorption. For instance, wheat bran fiber binds the minerals zinc, calcium, magnesium, and iron, reducing their absorption. A high-fiber diet is of particular concern when the overall diet is low in micronutrients, and in children because they have small stomachs and high nutrient needs. When mineral intake meets recommendations, a reasonable intake of high-fiber foods does not compromise mineral status.

When the diet is high in fiber, a larger volume of food must be consumed in order to meet energy requirements. This is generally beneficial because a high-fiber diet allows you to eat more food without gaining weight. However, for children who have small stomachs, consuming a diet that is very high in fiber may cause them to feel full before they have met all their nutrient needs.

HOW MUCH FIBER DO YOU NEED?

Most Americans do not eat enough fiber. The typical American diet contains only about 15 grams per day while the DRIs recommend a daily intake of 25 and 38 grams of fiber for young adult women and men, respectively. This recommendation is for total fiber, which includes dietary fiber and functional fiber. Dietary fiber is fiber that is found intact in plant foods. Functional fiber is fiber that has been isolated from foods and been shown to have beneficial physiological effects in humans. For example, the oat bran added to breads and breakfast cereals is functional fiber. Increasing your fiber intake means increasing your intake of plant foods that have only been minimally refined, such as fresh fruits and vegetables and whole grain products. Fiber intake can also be increased by consuming foods with added functional fiber such as cereal with added oat bran or flax seed. A system for estimating the fiber content of foods is shown in Table 3.2.

FACT BOX 3.2

Kellogg's Corn Flakes—A Health Food?

A belief that fiber is good for health is not new. Dr. John Harvey Kellogg believed that the bowel and the stomach were the cause of the majority of ailments. He believed that "autointoxication" was caused by eating meat; drinking alcohol and coffee; smoking; and overindulging in sex, spicy foods, and a host of other activities. Kellogg treated the rich and famous for a host of medical complaints at his Battle Creek Sanitarium (known as "the San"). He advocated vigorous exercise, sexual abstinence, and a high-fiber vegetarian diet, which, along with daily enemas, was designed to clean out the bowels. On March 7, 1897, Dr. Kellogg dished up the first serving of corn flakes at the San. These were an unsweetened addition to the diets of Dr. Kellogg's patients and were not the same corn flakes that you can buy today. The corn flakes we recognize today made their appearance in 1906. They were the brainchild of Dr. Kellogg's brother, Will Keith Kellogg, who added sugar to the recipe and began marketing them as a breakfast food. Dr. Kellogg was not supportive of this development and actually sued his brother in a failed attempt to keep the Kellogg name off of mass-produced breakfast cereals.

From: News of the Odd. "John Harvey Kellogg Serves Corn Flakes at the San (March 7, 1897)."
Available online at *http://www.newsoftheodd.com/article1016.html*.

Table 3.2 A System for Estimating the Fiber Content of a Diet

FOOD GROUP	FIBER PER SERVING		
	HIGH 4–5 GRAMS	**MEDIUM** 2 GRAMS	**LOW** 0.5–1 GRAM
Bread, Cereal, Rice, & Pasta Group			
Breads (1 slice)	—	Whole wheat Rye	White bread Bagel (1/2) Tortilla Roll (1/2) English muffin (1/2) Graham cracker
Cereals (1/2 cup)	All Bran Bran Buds 100% Bran flakes	40% Bran Shredded Wheat	Cheerios Rice Krispies
Rice and pasta (1/2 cup)	—	Whole wheat pasta Brown rice	Macaroni Pasta White rice
Fruit Group			
Fruits (1 medium or 1/2 cup)	Berries Prunes	Apple Apricot Banana Orange Raisins	Melon Canned fruit Juices
Vegetable Group			
Vegetables (1/2 cup)	Peas Broccoli Spinach	Green beans Carrots Eggplant Cabbage Potatoes with skin Corn	Asparagus Cauliflower Celery Lettuce Tomatoes Zucchini Peppers Potatoes without skin Onions
Dry Bean Group			
Beans (1/2 cup)	Beans: Pinto, red, kidney Black-eyed peas		

Adapted from Bright-See, E., Benda, C., Vartouhi, J., et al. "Development and testing of a dietary fibre exchange system." *Canadian Dietetic Association Journal* 47: 199–205, 1986; and Marlett, J. A. "Content and composition of dietary fiber in 117 frequently consumed foods." *Journal of the American Dietetic Association* 92: 175–186, 1992.

CONNECTIONS

Fiber cannot be digested by human enzymes in the gastrointestinal tract, so it is not absorbed into the body. Nonetheless, a diet high in fiber is important to health. Fiber is classified as either soluble or insoluble. Soluble fiber absorbs water and forms viscous solutions. Soluble fibers slow nutrient absorption and help reduce blood cholesterol levels. In the large intestine, soluble fibers can be broken down by intestinal bacteria, producing acids and gas, some of which can be absorbed into the body. Insoluble fibers are not broken down by intestinal bacteria but add bulk to intestinal contents. The added bulk stimulates intestinal motility and strengthens muscles in the colon. A high-fiber diet, when consumed with adequate fluid, reduces the risk of constipation and diverticulosis because stools are softer and less pressure is needed for defecation. A high-fiber diet may also reduce the risk of heart disease, diabetes, and colon cancer. Americans currently do not consume the recommended amounts of fiber.

4

Lipids

It is the cream that gives ice cream its smooth texture and the olive oil that gives Italian food its distinctive aroma and flavor. Creams, oils, and other fats (*lipid* is the chemical term for what we commonly call *fat*) contribute to the texture, flavor, and aroma of our food. While we crave them for their taste and texture, we are told to avoid them because too much fat, or at least too much of some types of fat, may increase our risk for heart disease, cancer, and obesity.

TYPES OF FATS

There are four types of lipids that are important in human nutrition: fatty acids, triglycerides, phospholipids, and sterols. Each has a different structure and function in the body.

Fatty Acids—Carbon Chains

Fatty acids consist of chains of carbon atoms linked together. Some fatty acids contain only a few carbons in this chain; others may

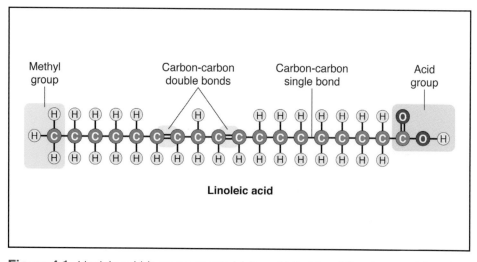

Figure 4.1 Linoleic acid is an unsaturated fatty acid that has 18 carbons and 2 carbon-carbon double bonds.

have 20 or more. Each carbon atom in the fatty acid chain forms four **chemical bonds** that can link it to as many as four other atoms. At one end of the chain, the omega end, the carbon atom is attached to its neighboring carbon and 3 hydrogen atoms to form a methyl group (CH_3); at the other end of the chain, the last carbon is part of an acid group (COOH). Each of the carbons in between is attached to 2 other carbons and up to 2 hydrogens. When each carbon in the fatty acid chain is bound to 2 hydrogens, it is a called a **saturated fatty acid** because the carbon chain is saturated with hydrogens. If the chain contains carbons that are not bound to 2 hydrogens, a double bond is formed between 2 carbons. Fatty acids containing one or more double bonds are called **unsaturated fatty acids** (Figure 4.1).

Saturated Fats

Saturated fatty acids or saturated fats are found primarily in animal foods such as meat, milk, and cheese. They are also found in palm oil, palm kernel oil, and coconut oil. These saturated vegetable oils are often called tropical oils because they are from plants common in tropical climates. They are used by the food industry in cereals, crackers, salad dressings, and cookies because these saturated fatty acids are more resistant to spoilage and therefore have a longer shelf life than unsaturated fats. It is important to recognize foods that are high in saturated fats because diets high in these are associated with an increased risk of heart disease.

Unsaturated Fats

Unsaturated fatty acids contain one or more unsaturated (double) bonds. Those that contain one double bond are called **mono-unsaturated** fatty acids. Oils that are high in monounsaturated fatty acids include olive, peanut, and canola oils. Fatty acids with more than one double bond in their carbon chains are called **polyunsaturated fatty acids**. Good sources of polyunsaturated fatty acids include corn, soybean, and safflower oils. Diets high in mono- and poly-unsaturated fats are associated with a reduced risk of heart disease.

Unsaturated fatty acids can be categorized based on the location of the first double bond in the carbon chain. If the first double bond occurs between the sixth and seventh carbons (from the omega, or CH_3, end) the fat is said to be an **omega-6 fatty acid**. The major omega-6 fatty acid in the American diet is linoleic acid, which is plentiful in vegetable oils. In the body, omega-6 fatty acids are important for growth, skin integrity, fertility, and maintaining red blood cell structure. Unsaturated fats with the first double bond between the third and fourth carbons, counting from the omega (CH_3) end of the chain are called **omega-3 fatty acids**. Alpha-linolenic acid, found in vegetable oils, and eicosapentaenoic acid (EPA) and docosahexaenoic acid (DHA), found in fish oils, are omega-3 fatty acids. Omega-3 fatty acids are important for the structure and function of cell membranes, particularly in the retina of the eye and the central nervous system. Diets high in omega-3 fatty acids may also be related to a reduced risk of heart disease. Supplements containing fish oils or purified omega-3 fatty acids are marketed to lower heart disease risk.

Because humans are not able to synthesize double bonds in the omega-6 and omega-3 positions, linoleic acid (omega-6) and alpha-linolenic acid (omega-3) are essential in the diet. They are needed to make other omega-6 and omega-3 fatty acids. For example, if the diet is low in linoleic acid, the omega-6 fatty acid arachidonic acid cannot be made and becomes a dietary essential. EPA and DHA are omega-3 fatty acids synthesized from alpha-linolenic acid.

If essential fatty acids are not consumed in adequate amounts, deficiency symptoms occur. The symptoms of an **essential fatty acid deficiency** include scaly, dry skin; liver abnormalities; poor healing of wounds; growth failure in infants; and impaired vision and hearing. Essential fatty acid deficiency is rare because the requirement for essential fatty acids is well below the amounts typically consumed.

Trans *Fats*

The position of the hydrogen atoms around the carbon-carbon double bonds in an unsaturated fatty acid affects its properties. Most unsaturated fatty acids have double bonds with both hydrogen atoms on the same side of the bond, the *cis* configuration. When the hydrogens are on opposite sides of the double bond, the fatty acid is a *trans* **fatty acid** (Figure 4.2). *Trans* fatty acids are found in small

---

FACT BOX 4.1

Fixing Infant Formulas

Docosahexaenoic acid (DHA) and arachidonic acid are important components of the central nervous system and the retina of the eye. DHA is an omega-3 fatty acid that can be made from alpha-linolenic acid, and arachidonic acid is an omega-6 fatty acid that can be made from linolenic acid. In adults, they can be made in the body in sufficient amounts to meet needs. But in infants, particularly premature infants, the rate at which these can be synthesized may be too slow to meet the need for optimal brain and retinal formation. This is not a problem in breast-fed infants because DHA and arachidonic acid are plentiful in breast milk. Recently, these acids have also been added to infant formulas.

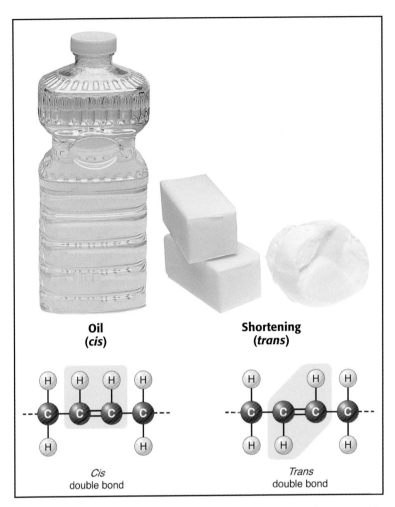

Figure 4.2 In a *cis* double bond, the hydrogens are on the same side of the double bond. In a *trans* double bond, the hydrogens are on opposite sides. During the hydrogenation of vegetable oils to make margarine and shortening, some of the *cis* bonds are converted to *trans*.

amounts in nature and are formed during the **hydrogenation** of vegetable oils. Hydrogenation is a process that adds hydrogen atoms to unsaturated fatty acids. This makes the fat more stable and more solid at room temperature. Diets high in *trans* fats are associated with an increased risk of heart disease.

Most Fatty Acids Are Found in Triglycerides

A triglyceride is made up of three fatty acids attached to a 3-carbon molecule called glycerol. Triglycerides make up most of the lipids in our food and in our bodies, and are usually what are referred to when the term *fat* is used. Triglycerides may contain any combination of fatty acids and it is their fatty acid composition that determines their taste, texture, physical characteristics, and health effects. When one fatty acid is attached, the molecule is called a monoglyceride and when two fatty acids are attached, it is a diglyceride.

Phospholipids Dissolve in Fat and Water

Phospholipids are important in foods and in the body because they allow water and oil to mix. They consist of a backbone of glycerol with two fatty acids and a phosphate group attached. A phosphate group is a chemical group containing the mineral phosphorous. It mixes well with water. In contrast, the fatty acid end of the molecule is soluble in fat. In foods, phospholipids act as **emulsifiers**, which break lipids into small droplets so they can mix with watery ingredients. For example, the phospholipid **lecithin** is used in salad dressings to keep the oil and water portions from separating. Phospholipids in the body are important in cell membranes. Cell membranes are made of two layers of phospholipid molecules in which the fatty acids are facing each other. This **lipid bilayer** allows an aqueous environment both inside and outside the cell with a lipid environment sandwiched between them.

Cholesterol and Other Sterols

Cholesterol is probably the best known of a type of lipid called a sterol. Sterols are lipids that have chemical rings as the basis of their structure. In the body, cholesterol is part of cell membranes and the insulating sheath that covers nerves. It is needed to synthesize vitamin D, bile acids, and a number of hormones, including the sex hormones. Although it is essential in the body, cholesterol is not a dietary essential because it is made in the liver. It is found only in animal foods; meats and dairy products contain cholesterol; egg yolks and organ meats are the richest sources. Plant foods do not contain cholesterol. A diet high in cholesterol can increase the risk of heart disease.

WHAT DO LIPIDS DO FOR US?

Lipids are involved in a number of functions in the body. They are needed to form body structures, regulate body processes, and provide energy. They are an important structural component of cells, particularly in the brain and nervous system. They are involved in regulation because they are needed to synthesize certain hormones, such as the sex hormones, and hormone-like molecules called **eicosanoids**, which help regulate blood clotting, blood pressure, immune function, and other body processes.[6] Omega-3 and omega-6 fatty acids make different eicosanoids; therefore, it is important to consume fats containing both omega-3 and omega-6 fatty acids in the diet.

Fat, as triglyceride, is an important energy source. When consumed in the diet, it can be used as an immediate source of energy or stored in the adipose tissue for future use. Because triglycerides are a concentrated energy source (9 cal/g), a large amount of energy can be stored in adipose tissue without a great increase in body size or weight. Adipose tissue also insulates the body from changes in temperature, and provides a cushion to protect against shock.

DIGESTING, ABSORBING, AND TRANSPORTING LIPIDS

Because most fats are large molecules that do not dissolve in water, they require special treatment during digestion, absorption, and transport through the body. Most of the digestion of lipids takes place in the small intestine through the action of enzymes called pancreatic **lipases**. Digestion and absorption of lipids are aided by **bile**. Bile is produced in the liver and stored in the gallbladder. It contains bile acids and helps break fat into small globules that can be accessed by enzymes. The enzymes break triglycerides into fatty acids, glycerol, and monoglycerides. The fatty acids and monoglycerides mix with bile and other lipids to form tiny droplets called micelles, which facilitate fat absorption.

After absorption into the cells lining the small intestine, small lipids, such as short and medium chain fatty acids, enter the blood and are transported to the liver. Larger fatty acids and monoglycerides are reassembled into triglycerides and then combined with cholesterol, phospholipids, and protein to form particles called **chylomicrons**. Chylomicrons are a type of **lipoprotein**. They are transported from the intestine via the **lymphatic system**. This transport route allows them to enter the bloodstream without first passing through the liver. As chylomicrons travel in the blood, triglycerides can be broken down into fatty acids and glycerol, which enter the surrounding cells. What remains of the chylomicron goes to the liver. Once at the liver, the remnants of chylomicrons as well as triglycerides and cholesterol synthesized in the liver are incorporated into lipoprotein particles called **very-low-density lipoproteins (VLDLs)**. VLDLs transport lipids from the liver and deliver triglycerides to body cells. As VLDLs travel in the blood and triglycerides are removed, VLDLs are transformed into a particle that can either be returned to the liver or used to form lipoproteins called **low-density lipoproteins (LDLs)**. LDLs deliver cholesterol to body cells. For LDLs to be taken up by cells, the LDL particle must bind to a protein on the cell membrane, called an LDL receptor. High levels of LDLs in the blood are associated with an increased risk for heart disease. Cholesterol that is not used by cells is returned to the liver by **high-density lipoproteins (HDLs)**. High levels of HDLs in the blood are associated with a reduction in heart disease risk.

FACT BOX 4.2

Evidence of a Fatty Meal

Chylomicrons enter your blood from the gastrointestinal tract. The more fat you eat in a meal, the more chylomicrons appear in the blood. If you have a blood sample taken after eating a fatty meal, your blood plasma will look as white as milk because of the large number of fatty chylomicron droplets floating around. A few hours later, cells will have taken up the fat and the plasma will be a clear yellowish color again.

LIPID METABOLISM: USING AND STORING FAT

The fatty acids we consume in our diets can be used to produce ATP via cellular respiration. For this to occur, the carbon chains of fatty acids must first be broken into 2-carbon units that form acetyl CoA. Acetyl CoA can then be metabolized by aerobic metabolism to generate ATP. After the body's immediate need for energy is met, remaining fatty acids can be stored in the adipose tissue as triglycerides. Stored triglycerides are broken down and reformed depending on the immediate energy needs of the body.

When the diet contains enough calories to meet needs, the net amount of stored triglycerides in adipose tissue does not change and body weight remains constant. When less energy is consumed than is needed, the body releases stored triglycerides to be used for fuel and weight is lost. When excess energy is consumed as fat, the fatty acids are transported directly to the adipose tissue for storage. If excess energy is consumed as carbohydrates or protein, these must first go to the liver, where they can be used, although inefficiently, to synthesize fatty acids. These are then assembled into triglycerides, and delivered to the adipose tissue for storage. As more fat is stored, adipose tissue cells get bigger. They can increase in weight by about 50 times, and new fat cells can be made when existing cells reach their maximum size.

FACT BOX 4.3

Brown and Goldstein

In 1985, Drs. Michael Brown and Joseph Goldstein were awarded the Nobel Prize in Medicine for their discovery of LDL receptors. These are proteins, present on the surface of cells, that act as docks where LDL cholesterol attaches to the cell and can move inside to deliver its cargo of cholesterol. Brown and Goldstein made their discovery by studying people with a genetic condition in which the LDL receptors are absent. Without LDL receptors, the cholesterol cannot leave the blood. People with this condition have blood cholesterol levels that are 6 times higher than normal and suffer from clogged arteries in childhood and adolescence.

LIPIDS AND HEART DISEASE

Diets high in saturated fat and cholesterol may increase the risk of developing heart disease, in particular, **atherosclerosis**. Atherosclerosis is a type of heart disease in which a fatty substance called plaque builds up in arteries. Plaque causes an artery to narrow and lose its elasticity. The buildup of plaque can become so great that it completely blocks the artery, or a blood clot that forms around the plaque can break loose and block a smaller artery elsewhere. When blood can no longer move through a blood vessel, the cells it supplies are starved for oxygen and die. If an artery in the heart is blocked, heart muscle cells die, resulting in a heart attack or myocardial infarction. If the blood flow to the brain is interrupted, brain cells die and a stroke results.

There are many factors that affect the risk of developing atherosclerosis. Risk increases with increasing age and is higher in men at a younger age. Other conditions, including high blood pressure, diabetes, obesity, high blood LDL cholesterol, and low blood HDL cholesterol, also increase the risk (Table 4.1). Lifestyle factors such as lack of exercise, stress, cigarette smoking, and a diet high in saturated fat, *trans* fat, and cholesterol also increase risk. On the other hand, regular exercise decreases risk by promoting the maintenance of a healthy body weight, reducing the risk of diabetes, increasing HDL cholesterol, and reducing blood pressure. Diets high in omega-3 fatty acids help to reduce LDL cholesterol levels and help to prevent the growth of atherosclerotic plaque by affecting blood

---

FACT BOX 4.4

Heart Disease Statistics

It is estimated that 61.8 million Americans have one or more forms of cardiovascular disease. These diseases cause 1 out of every 2.5 deaths. With new emphasis on prevention, currently about 12 million Americans are taking a class of cholesterol-lowing drugs called statins in order to reduce their risk of heart disease. Statins work by reducing cholesterol synthesis in the liver.

From: American Heart Association Cardiovascular Disease Statistics. Available online at
    http://www.americanheart.org/presenter.jhtml?identifier=4478).

Table 4.1 Factors That Affect Heart Disease Risk

AGE: Risk increases with increasing age.			
SEX: Males have a higher risk until age 65, then risks do not differ between the sexes.			
DISEASE FACTORS:			
Diabetes: Fasting blood sugar greater than 126 mg/100 ml			
High blood pressure: Greater than 140/90			
Obesity: Body mass index greater than 27			
High blood lipid levels:			
	Low Risk	**Moderate Risk**	**High Risk**
Total cholesterol (mg/100 ml)	< 200	200–239	≥ 240
LDL cholesterol (mg/100 ml)	< 100	130–159	≥ 160
HDL (mg/100 ml)	≥ 60	40–59	≤ 40
LIFESTYLE:			
Risk is increased by:			
Cigarette smoking			
Stress			
Sedentary lifestyle			
Risk is decreased by:			
Regular exercise			
DIET:			
Risk is increased by:			
High total fat intake			
High saturated fat intake			
High cholesterol intake			
High intake of *trans* fat			
Risk is decreased by:			
High intake of omega-3 fatty acids			
High fiber intake			
High intake of fruits and vegetables			
High intake of antioxidant nutrients such as vitamin E			

clotting, blood pressure, and immune function.[7] Diets high in mono-unsaturated fats, such as those consumed in Mediterranean countries where olive oil is commonly used, also reduce LDL cholesterol and keep HDL levels high. Diets high in plant foods are associated with a lower risk of heart disease. This may be due to the increased fiber, antioxidant, and **phytochemical** content of these diets. Phytochemicals are compounds found in plants, many of which have health-promoting properties. Moderate alcohol consumption has also been shown to lower risk by reducing stress and raising HDL cholesterol levels.

HOW MUCH AND WHAT KIND OF FAT DO WE NEED?

Fat is an essential nutrient. We need to consume enough of the essential fatty acids to prevent deficiencies; the DRIs have made specific recommendations for the amounts of essential omega-6 and omega-3 fatty acids (see Appendix B). In addition to the role of specific fats in the body, fat is an energy-yielding nutrient. To meet calorie needs and balance the amounts of the carbohydrate, protein, and fat in our diets, the DRIs recommend that American adults consume between 20% and 35% of their calories as fat. The current fat intake in the United States is about 33% of calories.[2] This is close to the upper end of the DRI recommendations and slightly above the Daily Value recommendation on food labels of 30% or less of calories from fat.

In terms of health, the type of fat consumed is as important as the amount. Diets high in mono- and polyunsaturated fats are associated with a low risk of heart disease and diets high in saturated fat, cholesterol, and *trans* fat are associated with a high risk. Although specific recommendations have not been set for the amount of cholesterol, saturated fat, and *trans* fat in the diet, intake of these should be kept to a minimum because the risk of heart disease increases with higher intake.

CONNECTIONS

Lipids, commonly called fats, consist of fatty acids, triglycerides, phospholipids, and sterols. Fatty acids can be either saturated or unsaturated. Saturated fats are most abundant in animal foods. Diets high in saturated fats are associated with an increased risk of heart disease. Unsaturated fats include mono- and polyunsaturated fats. They are found primarily in plant foods and diets high in these reduce the risk of heart disease. *Trans* fats are a type of unsaturated fat produced during a process called hydrogenation that is used to make margarine from vegetable oils. Diets high in *trans* fat increase the risk of heart disease. Most of the fat in our diets and in our bodies is made up of triglycerides, which consist of 3 fatty acids attached to a molecule of glycerol. Triglycerides are a major energy source for the

---

FACT BOX 4.5

How Much Fat Is in Your Diet?

The DRIs recommend that you consume between 20% and 35% of your energy from fat. The Daily Values recommend 30% or less, but how do you know what percentage of the energy in your diet is from fat? To find out, you need to know how many calories and how many grams of fat you eat each day. You can get this information by using a diet analysis computer program or food composition tables. Knowing that fat provides 9 calories per gram allows you to do the following calculation:

- Multiply the grams of fat by 9 calories per gram

    Grams fat x 9 calories/gram fat = Calories from fat

- Divide calories from fat by total calories in the diet and multiply by 100 to express as a percent

$$\frac{\text{Calories from fat}}{\text{Total calories}} \text{ x } 100 = \text{Percent calories from fat}$$

For example:

If your diet contains 2,000 calories and 62 g of fat

    62 g of fat x 9 cal/g = 558 calories from fat

$$\frac{558 \text{ calories from fat}}{2,000 \text{ calories}} \text{ x } 100 = 28\% \text{ of energy (calories) from fat}$$

body, providing 9 calories per gram. Cholesterol is a type of sterol found only in animal foods. High intakes may increase the risk of heart disease. In the body, lipids are transported through the blood in particles called lipoproteins, which include chylomicrons, VLDLs, LDLs, and HDLs. High blood levels of LDLs increase the risk of heart disease, whereas high levels of HDLs decrease the risk. Recommendations for a healthy diet suggest that you consume between 20% and 35% of energy from fat and limit the amount of saturated fat, *trans* fat, and cholesterol in your diet.

5

Protein

Strength, health, and vitality—all of these attributes are associated with protein. Body builders eat it to bulk up their muscles, fashion models eat it to make their skin glow, and manufacturers add it to shampoos to strengthen hair. What is this wondrous substance? Does it really do all these things for us?

WHAT IS PROTEIN?

The proteins that make up our muscles, skin, and hair are large molecules made of chainlike strands of smaller molecules called amino acids. Unlike carbohydrates and lipids, which are made of only carbon, hydrogen, and oxygen atoms, proteins also contain the element nitrogen. The nitrogen is in a chemical group called an amino group (NH_2) that is part of the structure of each amino acid. Amino acids also contain an acid group (COOH) and a side chain that varies in structure. Amino acids are the building blocks of proteins. There are 20 different amino acids commonly found in proteins; they all have different side chains. Some of the amino acids found in protein can be made in the body, usually by moving the amino group from an amino acid to a carbon chain to form a different amino acid. Others cannot be made by the human body. These **essential amino acids** must be consumed in the diet. Some amino acids are conditionally essential; that is, they are essential only under certain conditions. For example, the amino acid tyrosine can be made in the body from the essential amino acid phenylalanine. However, if phenylalanine is deficient, tyrosine must be consumed in the diet.

To make a protein, chains of amino acids are linked together by peptide bonds. Two amino acids linked together form a dipeptide; three form a tripeptide; many together constitute a polypeptide. The final protein consists of one or more polypeptide chains that fold over on themselves to form a complex three-dimensional shape. Different polypeptides contain different amino acids in different proportions bound together in a specific order. Variations in the number, proportion, and order of amino acids allow for an infinite number of different polypeptide and protein structures. The order

---

FACT BOX 5.1

What Is a Phenylketonuric?

Have you ever read your can of diet soda? If you look closely, you will see a warning that says "Phenylketonurics: Contains phenylalanine." Should you be worried? What is a phenylketonuric? A phenylketonuric is someone with a genetic disease called phenylketonuria. These people have a genetic defect that prevents them from breaking down the amino acid phenylalanine. As a result, a by-product called phenylketone accumulates in their blood and can cause brain damage. To stay healthy, individuals with phenylketonuria must eat a diet low in phenylalanine. Diet soda made with the artificial sweetener aspartame contains phenylalanine because aspartame is made of two amino acids: aspartic acid and phenylalanine. The warning on diet soda serves to alert people with phenylketonuria that the soda, which would normally not be a source of any amino acids, contains phenylalanine.

of the amino acids in a polypeptide chain determines the three-dimensional shape the final protein will have; this, in turn, affects the protein's function (Figure 5.1).

WHAT DO PROTEINS DO?

Proteins serve many different functions in the body. They provide the structure of hair and nails. They form the framework of bones into which minerals are deposited. The proteins in muscles form their structure and allow them to contract. Protein hormones help regulate body processes and enzymes made of protein speed up the rate of chemical reactions in the body. Proteins are also an integral part of cell membranes, where they help transport materials in and out of cells and help cells communicate with one another. Proteins in our blood help transport materials throughout the body, regulate the distribution of water in the body, and keep body fluids at the right acidity. Proteins produced by our immune system help protect us from disease. If necessary, body proteins can also be broken down to provide energy.

DIGESTING AND ABSORBING PROTEIN

Protein that is consumed in the diet must be broken down in order to be absorbed into the body. Protein digestion begins in the stomach, where hydrochloric acid unfolds the polypeptide chains that make up a protein to allow the protein-digesting enzyme **pepsin** to begin breaking these large molecules into shorter polypeptides and amino acids. In the intestine, the polypeptides are broken into smaller peptides by enzymes secreted by the pancreas. Small peptides are broken into single amino acids by enzymes found on the surface of and inside the cells lining the small intestine.

Amino acids are absorbed by several different energy-requiring transport systems. Amino acids with similar structures share the same transport system and therefore compete with each other for absorption. If there is an excess of any one of the amino acids sharing a transport system, more of that amino acid will be absorbed, slowing the absorption of the other amino acids.

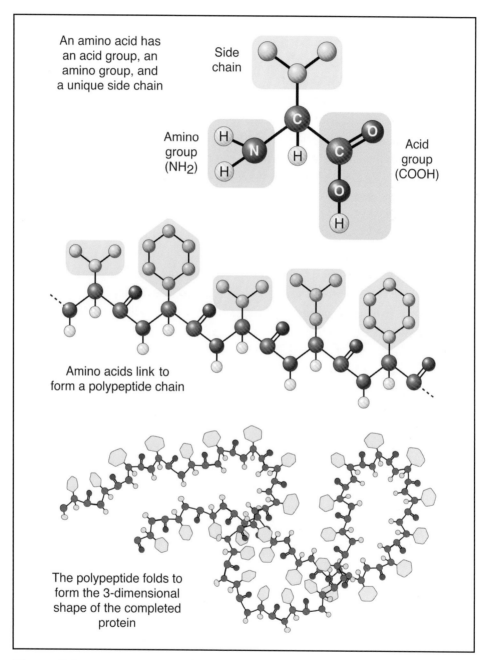

An amino acid has an acid group, an amino group, and a unique side chain

Side chain

Amino group (NH$_2$)

Acid group (COOH)

Amino acids link to form a polypeptide chain

The polypeptide folds to form the 3-dimensional shape of the completed protein

Figure 5.1 Amino acids are linked together to form polypeptides, which fold to form proteins.

For this reason, taking supplements of a single amino acid can block the absorption of others sharing the same transport system.

PROTEIN METABOLISM: MAKING AND BREAKING PROTEINS

Once the amino acids from dietary protein have been absorbed, they become available to make the proteins needed by the body, to make other molecules that contain nitrogen, or to provide energy.

Making Body Proteins

Body proteins are synthesized from amino acids—some of these come from protein consumed in the diet and some come from the breakdown of body proteins. Of the approximately 300 grams of protein synthesized by the body each day, only about 100 grams are made of amino acids from the diet. The other 200 grams are made from amino acids recycled from protein broken down in the body.

The instructions for making body proteins are contained in DNA in the nucleus of cells. A stretch of DNA that provides the blueprint for the structure of a protein is called a gene. To make a protein, the information from a gene is copied into a molecule of RNA. The RNA takes this information from the nucleus to structures called ribosomes located in the cell's cytoplasm. At the ribosome, the information in RNA is translated into the sequence of amino acids that makes up the protein (Figure 5.2). Which proteins are made and when they are made is regulated. For example, if a protein is needed by the body, the process of protein synthesis is turned on. For the process to be completed, all the amino acids needed for that protein must be available. If one is missing, protein synthesis stops until the amino acid is provided. If the missing amino acid is a nonessential amino acid, it can be made by the body. If the missing amino acid is an essential amino acid, the body must break down other body proteins to obtain it. The essential amino acid present in the shortest supply relative to need is called the limiting amino acid, because lack of this amino acid limits the ability to make the protein.

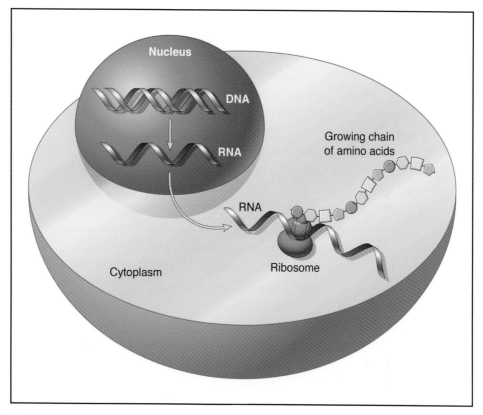

Figure 5.2 To synthesize a protein, the information in DNA is transcribed into a molecule of RNA. The RNA takes the information to the ribosomes in the cytoplasm of the cell, where it dictates the sequence of amino acids in a protein.

Making Nonprotein Molecules

Amino acids are also used to make other molecules that contain nitrogen. These include the units that make up DNA and RNA, the high-energy molecule ATP, the skin pigment melanin, a number of **neurotransmitters**, and histamine, which causes blood vessels to dilate.

Using Protein for Energy

Carbohydrates and fat are more efficient energy sources than protein, but when the diet provides more protein than the body needs, some of the dietary protein can be used to produce energy. Protein is also used as an energy source when the diet does not contain enough energy to meet needs. In this situation, body proteins are broken down into amino acids to supply energy.

To be used for energy, the nitrogen-containing amino group must be removed from amino acids. The remaining carbon compound can then enter the citric acid cycle to produce ATP or be used to make glucose via gluconeogenesis. Body proteins can provide energy and glucose in times of need, but using them for this purpose also robs the body of functional proteins.

HOW DOES PROTEIN INTAKE AFFECT HEALTH?

Although a protein deficiency is uncommon in the United States, in developing nations, concerns about inadequate protein are very real. Diets lacking protein are often deficient in energy as well, but a pure protein deficiency can occur when protein needs are high and food choices are very low in protein. The term **protein-energy malnutrition (PEM)** is used to refer to the continuum of conditions ranging from pure protein deficiency, called **kwashiorkor**, to energy deficiency, called **marasmus** (Figure 5.3).

The word *kwashiorkor* means "the disease that the first child gets when the second child is born." It occurs at this time because, when a new baby is born, the first child no longer is fed high-protein breast milk but rather must try to meet his or her needs by consuming the local diet. The symptoms include reduced growth, increased susceptibility to infection, changes in hair color, dry flaking skin, and bloated bellies. Children with kwashiorkor have bloated bellies because fat and fluid accumulate in their abdomens. Although kwashiorkor is often thought of as a disease of children, it is also seen in ill adults who have high-protein needs due to infection or trauma and a low-protein intake because they are unable to eat.

The word *marasmus* means "to waste away." The lack of energy causes growth to slow or stop, body fat stores to be depleted, and muscles to shrink, making the body appear emaciated. It is the form of malnutrition that occurs with eating disorders. It has devastating effects in infants and children because adequate energy is essential

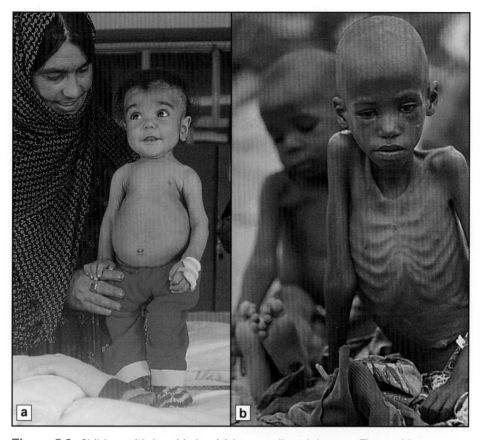

Figure 5.3 Children with kwashiorkor (a) have swollen abdomens. Those with marasmus (b) exhibit severe wasting of their body fat and muscle. Both diseases are forms of malnutrition.

for growth and brain development. It is seen in the United States in patients with cancer or AIDS as well as in individuals who are starving themselves due to an eating disorder.

An excess intake of protein has no immediate effects other than increasing fluid needs. The extra fluid is needed to excrete the additional nitrogen that is removed when amino acids are broken down. It has been suggested that the long-term consumption of diets high in protein may have a negative effect on kidney function. The other concern associated with high-protein diets is that they are high in animal foods, which are high in saturated fat and cholesterol and may therefore increase the risk of heart disease.

HOW MUCH PROTEIN DO YOU NEED?

The DRIs recommend 0.8 grams of protein per kilogram of body weight for adults; this is about 72 grams per day for a 200-pound man. A typical American diet exceeds this, providing about 100 grams daily. This amount of protein, however, is well within the DRI recommendation that protein account for 10% to 35% of calories from protein.

Protein needs per kilogram of body weight are higher for children, teens, and pregnant women to ensure that they have enough protein to allow for growth. Lactation also increases the body's protein demand because the milk produced and secreted is high in protein. Extreme stresses on the body such as infections, fevers, burns, and surgery increase protein losses and therefore increase dietary needs. Endurance and strength sports may also increase protein needs. In endurance events such as marathons, protein is used for energy and to maintain blood glucose, so athletes involved in these activities may benefit from 1.2 to 1.4 grams of protein per kilogram per day. Strength athletes who require amino acids to synthesize new muscle proteins may benefit from 1.6 to 1.7 grams per kilogram per day. This amount, however, is not much more than the amount contained in the diets of typical American athletes. For example, a 190-pound man consuming 3,000 calories, 18% of which comes from protein, would be consuming 135 grams, or 1.6 grams of protein per kg body weight. If the diet is adequate in energy, this amount of protein can easily be obtained from the diet without protein or amino acid supplements.

VEGETARIAN DIETS

When we think of protein, we usually think of animal foods like beef, chicken, milk, and cheese. However, plant foods such as soybeans, sunflower seeds, almonds, and rice also provide protein. Much of the world survives primarily on plant proteins—mostly out of necessity because animal foods are typically more expensive and less available. In affluent societies where animal foods are available, some people may still choose to consume only plant proteins for health, religious, ethical, or environmental reasons. The strictest of these vegetarian diets eliminates all animal foods—these are called **vegan** diets. Other vegetarian diets allow some animal foods. For example, semivegetarians avoid only certain types of red meat, fish, or poultry; lacto-ovo vegetarians eat no animal flesh but do eat eggs and dairy products; and lacto vegetarians avoid animal flesh and eggs but do consume dairy products.

FACT BOX 5.2

Do Vegetarian Diets Help the Environment?

One of the reasons people choose to adopt vegetarian diets is concern about the environment. It takes more energy and resources to raise animals than it does to grow plants. For every 100 calories of plant material a cow eats, only 10 calories are stored in the cow and can be consumed by humans.[a] In the United States, 1 pound of pork provides 1,000 to 2,000 calories in the diet and costs 14,000 calories to produce. Worldwide, 38% of the total grain produced is fed to chickens, pigs, and cows. Although it is more efficient to take animals out of this equation, the solution is not so simple. If animals are used wisely, they can add to the food supply, rather than waste grain that humans might eat. The natural ecosystems of the Earth include both plants and animals. Animals can live on land that will not support crops and eat plants that will not nourish humans. Eliminating animal products entirely would reduce both the variety of food and the nutrient content of the human diet. A better solution is to develop sustainable agricultural systems in which cattle and sheep would eat only from grazing lands that are unsuitable for growing crops, rather than be fed grains that can be consumed by humans. Both plants and animals are essential for a diversified ecosystem, and both plant and animal foods make valuable contributions to the human diet.

a Raven, P.H., Berg, L.R., and Johnson, G.B. *Environment,* 3rd ed. Philadelphia: Harcourt College Publishers, 2001.

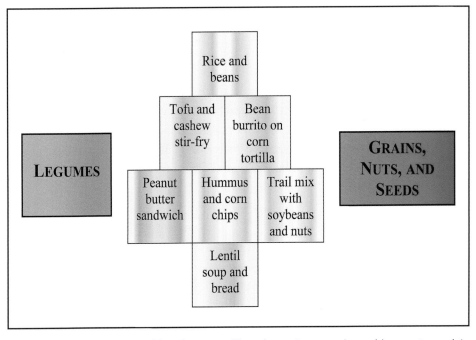

Figure 5.4 A meal that combines legumes with grains, nuts, or seeds provides more complete protein than either of these plant protein sources provides alone.

Protein Complementation

Vegetarians are able to meet their protein needs by consuming a mix of plant proteins that provides all of the amino acids needed to build body proteins. Generally, the proteins in animal foods provide a mixture of amino acids that is closer to body needs than plant proteins do. Therefore, animal proteins are said to be of higher **protein quality** than plant proteins. Plant proteins are limited in one or more essential amino acids, so to get all of the essential amino acids and thus meet protein needs, plant foods with complementary combinations of amino acids must be consumed. This is the principle of protein complementation—combining foods containing proteins with different limiting amino acids in order to improve the protein quality of the diet as a whole. The amino acids that are most often limited in plant proteins are lysine, methionine, cysteine, and tryptophan. As a general rule, legumes such as chickpeas, black beans, and lentils are deficient in methionine and cysteine but high in lysine. Grains, nuts, and seeds are deficient in lysine but high in methionine and cysteine. Corn is deficient in lysine and tryptophan but is a good source of methionine. By combining plant proteins with complementary amino acid patterns, all essential amino acids requirements can be met (Figure 5.4). Although it is not necessary to consume complementary proteins at each meal, the entire day's diet should include proteins from a variety of plant sources in order to satisfy the daily need for amino acids.[8]

Pros and Cons of Vegetarian Diets

Vegetarian diets can be a healthy alternative to the typical diet. Because they limit animal foods, they are lower in saturated fat and cholesterol and because they tend to be higher in grains, legumes, vegetables, and fruits, they are higher in fiber, vitamins, minerals, and phytochemicals.[9] Vegetarians have been shown to have lower risks for obesity, diabetes, cardiovascular disease, high blood pressure, and some types of cancer.[8,10]

Despite their benefits, vegetarian diets can be deficient in certain vitamins and minerals. Diets that exclude dairy products may be deficient in calcium and vitamin D. Diets that exclude red meat may be low in iron and zinc because red meats are the best sources of these minerals. Vegan diets, which exclude all animal foods, will

---

FACT BOX 5.3

Super Soy

In general, animal proteins are of higher quality than plant proteins. An exception is soy protein, which can meet protein needs as well as any animal protein. In addition to its high-quality protein, soy may have some other benefits. It has been found to reduce the risk of heart disease and there is evidence that it may also reduce the risk of certain cancers and alleviate some menopausal symptoms. To get these benefits, however, you need to eat 10 to 25 grams a day—the equivalent of a soy burger or a quarter cup of roasted soybeans.

be deficient in vitamin B_{12} because this vitamin is found almost exclusively in animal products. Nutrient deficiencies are a particular concern if vegetarian diets are consumed by those with increased needs such as small children or pregnant women, but vitamin B_{12} deficiency is a concern for anyone eating a vegan diet.

Choosing a Vegetarian Diet

Vegetarians can meet their needs by modifying their selections from the Food Guide Pyramid. The food choices and recommended number of servings from the grains, vegetables, and fruits, found in the bottom two levels of the pyramid, are the same as for non-vegetarians. The groups in the next level of the Pyramid (meat and milk) include foods of animal origin. Vegetarians can meet their protein needs by choosing 2 to 3 servings of dry beans, nuts, seeds, eggs, and meat substitutes. Lacto vegetarians (those who consume dairy products) should also consume 2 to 3 servings from the milk group. Vegans should consume milk substitutes fortified with calcium and vitamin D, or other foods high in these nutrients. To obtain adequate vitamin B_{12}, vegans must take B_{12} supplements or use products fortified with vitamin B_{12}.

CONNECTIONS

Protein in the diet provides the building blocks for body proteins. Proteins are made of chainlike strands of amino acids. Some amino acids are dietary essentials and some can be made in the body. The order and number of amino acids in the chain is unique to each protein and determines the final structure of the protein, which in turn determines its function. DNA in the nucleus of body cells provides the information needed to synthesize proteins from amino acids. Body proteins provide structure and also serve regulatory roles as enzymes, hormones, and transport molecules. They function in the immune system, muscle contraction, and fluid and acid balance. Protein can also be metabolized to provide energy. Amino acids are used to synthesize a number of small nitrogen-containing molecules. The typical American diet provides plenty of protein for most people. A diet that is deficient in protein leads to protein-energy malnutrition, which includes kwashiorkor and marasmus. These are significant health problems in developing countries. Protein in the diet is found in both animal and plant foods. The protein in animal foods provides a mix of amino acids that better meets human needs and is therefore said to be high-quality protein. By combining lower-quality protein from different plant sources, the protein quality of a vegitarian diet can be improved and can meet protein needs. Vegetarian diets may, however, be low in calcium, vitamin D, iron, zinc, or vitamin B_{12}. Vegetarians can choose a healthy diet by modifying their selections from the Food Guide Pyramid.

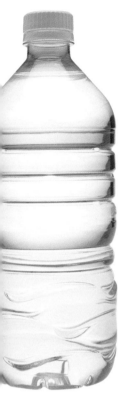

6

Water

Water—the elixir of life. Without it, you cannot survive more than about four days. It is a small **inorganic** molecule made up of one oxygen and two hydrogen atoms, but gram for gram, we need more water than carbohydrate, fat, or protein. A deficiency of water will cause symptoms faster than a deficiency of any other nutrient. Even minor changes in the amount and distribution of body water can be life-threatening. For example, days and even weeks without some vitamins and minerals will not cause deficiency symptoms, but an hour of exercise in a hot environment can cause symptoms that are due to too little water. If you do not replace this water, you may begin to experience severe symptoms such as nausea, dizziness, and weakness.

WHAT DOES WATER DO?
The human body is about 60% water—this water allows for the transport of nutrients, provides structure, is needed in chemical reactions in the body, and regulates body temperature.

Water Transports Substances

Water bathes the cells of the body and serves as a transport medium to deliver substances to cells and remove wastes. For example, blood, which is 90% water, transports oxygen, nutrients, hormones, drugs, and other substances to cells. It then carries carbon dioxide and other waste products away from the cells. Water in urine helps eliminate wastes from the body.

Water Provides Structure and Protection

Water is a part of the structure of a number of molecules, including glycogen and proteins. It also makes up most of the volume of body cells. Muscle is about 75% water and even bone is 25% water. Water helps protect the body by serving as a lubricant and cleanser. Watery tears lubricate the eyes and wash away dirt, synovial fluid lubricates the joints, and saliva lubricates the mouth, making it easier to chew and swallow food. Water inside the eyeballs and spinal cord also protects the body by acting as a cushion against shock.

Water Is Needed for Chemical Reactions

Water is involved in numerous chemical reactions throughout the body. One way in which it is involved is to serve as the medium in which all of the body's metabolic reactions occur. Water is an ideal **solvent** for many substances because the two ends of the water molecule have different electrical charges—one end is positive and one end is negative. This property allows water to surround other charged molecules and disperse them. For example, table salt, which dissolves in water, consists of a positively charged sodium ion bound to a negatively charged chloride ion. When placed in water, the sodium and chloride ions move apart because the positively charged sodium ion is attracted to the negative end of the water molecule and the negatively charged chloride ion is attracted to the positive end.

Water also participates directly in a number of chemical reactions, many of which are involved in energy production. The addition of water to a large molecule can break it into two smaller ones.

Likewise, the removal of a water molecule can join two molecules together. Some of the reactions in which water participates help maintain the proper level of acidity in the body. Acid balance in the body is regulated by a number of different systems. These include chemical reactions in body fluids, gas exchange at the lungs, and filtration by the kidneys. Water plays an important role in each of these, in some cases by participating directly in a chemical reaction and in other cases by helping to transport substances to the lungs or kidneys.

Water Regulates Body Temperature

The metabolic reactions that are essential for life generate heat. To maintain body temperature in the range that is compatible with health and life, this heat must be eliminated. Likewise, in a cold environment, heat must be conserved so body temperature does not drop too low.

The water in blood helps regulate body temperature by increasing or decreasing the amount of heat lost at the body surface. When body temperature starts to rise, the blood vessels in the skin dilate, causing blood to flow close to the surface of the body where it can release some of the heat to the environment. This is the reason your skin becomes red in hot weather or during strenuous activity. In a cold environment, the opposite occurs. The blood vessels in the skin constrict, restricting the flow of blood near the surface and conserving body heat.

The most obvious way that water helps regulate body temperature is through the evaporation of sweat. When body temperature increases, the brain triggers the sweat glands in the skin to produce sweat, which is mostly water. As the sweat evaporates from the skin, heat is lost, cooling the body.

HOW DO YOU GET WATER INTO THE BODY?

Water in the body comes from water in the diet—mostly as water itself and other fluids but also from solid food (Figure 6.1). For example, low-fat milk is 90% water, apples are about 85% water, and roast beef is about 50% water. A small amount of water is

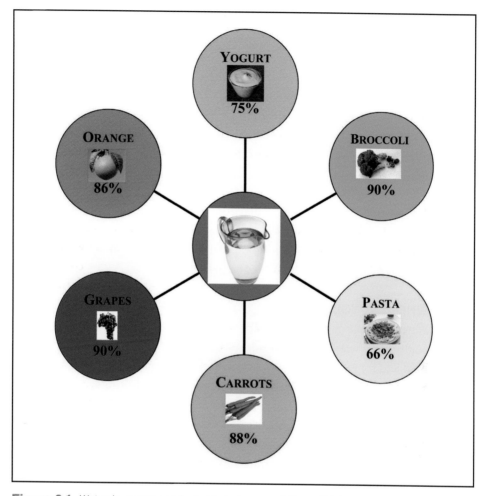

Figure 6.1 Water is consumed in fluids but many of the solid foods consumed in the diet are also good sources of water. The percentages in each circle indicate the amount of that food's weight that is water.

generated inside the body by metabolism, but this is not significant in meeting body water needs.

Water is absorbed from the gastrointestinal tract by osmosis. **Osmosis** is the movement of water across a membrane from an area with a low concentration of dissolved substances to an area with a high concentration of dissolved substances. The volume of water and the density of nutrients consumed with it influence the rate of absorption. Consuming a large volume of water increases its rate of absorption. Water consumed alone will easily move from the intestine into the blood, where the concentration of **solutes** is higher. When water is consumed with meals, absorption is slower because the concentration of dissolved substances in the intestine is higher. As the nutrients from the meal move from the intestine into the plasma, the solute concentration in the intestine decreases and water moves by osmosis toward the area with the highest solute concentration.

About 1.7 liters of water enters the GI tract each day from the diet. Another 7 liters comes from saliva and other gastrointestinal secretions. Most of this fluid is absorbed in the small intestine but a small amount is also absorbed in the colon.

WHERE IN YOUR BODY IS WATER LOCATED?

Water is found in varying proportions in all the tissues of the body. Some of this water is found inside cells and is known as **intracellular fluid** and some is located outside cells and is known as **extracellular fluid**. Extracellular fluid accounts for about one-third of total body water and is made up primarily of the water in blood plasma and the fluid between cells, called **interstitial fluid**. Interstitial fluid makes up about three-fourths of the extracellular fluid and plasma about one-fourth. Other extracellular fluids include lymph and fluids in cavities, such as that inside the lumen of the GI tract, the eyes, joints, and spinal cord.

Dissolved substances such as sodium, chloride, and potassium (as well as magnesium, calcium, and many other small molecules) play an important role in regulating where the water is located in the body. Water can move freely between the different body compartments in a direction that will equalize the concentration of dissolved particles. Therefore, it is the concentrations of dissolved substances that determine the distribution of water among the various compartments. For example, if the concentration of sodium in the blood is high, water from the interstitial fluid is drawn into the blood, diluting the sodium. Sodium and other dissolved substances help maintain fluid balance within the body by helping to keep water within a particular compartment. The concentration of dissolved substances is also important in regulating the total amount of body water.

BALANCING WATER IN WITH WATER OUT

Water cannot be stored. Therefore, to maintain adequate water in the body, water intake and excretion must be regulated. Intake is stimulated by thirst and losses are precisely regulated by the kidneys.

Thirst

How do you know when you need water? The need to consume water or other fluids is signaled by the sensation of thirst. Thirst is triggered both by sensations in the mouth and signals from the brain. The mouth becomes dry because less water is available for saliva. The thirst center in the brain senses a decrease in the amount of fluid in blood and an increase in the concentration of dissolved substances in this fluid. Together, the feeling of a dry mouth and signals from the brain cause the sensation of thirst and motivate us to drink.

Thirst is not a perfect regulator of water intake, however. Feeling thirsty does not mean that you will take a drink. Also, the sensation of thirst often lags behind the need for water. For example, athletes exercising in hot weather lose water rapidly but do not experience intense thirst until they have lost so much body water that their physical performance is compromised.[11] In addition, thirst is quenched almost as soon as fluid is consumed and often long before adequate body water is restored. Because people cannot and do not always respond adequately to thirst, water loss from the body is regulated by the kidneys to prevent dehydration.

Water Losses

Water is lost from the body in urine and feces, through evaporation from the lungs and skin, and in sweat. A typical young man loses about 2.75 liters of water daily through urine, feces, and evaporation. This amount must be replaced through consumption of food and fluids in order to maintain water balance.

Typical urine output is 1 to 2 liters per day, but this varies depending on the amount of fluid consumed and the amount of waste to be excreted. Some of the waste products that must be excreted in urine include **urea** and other nitrogen-containing products from protein breakdown, **ketones** from fat breakdown, phosphates, sulfates, electrolytes, and other minerals. The amount of urea that must be excreted is increased when dietary protein intake or body protein breakdown is increased. Ketone excretion is increased when body fat is broken down. The amount of sodium that must be excreted is increased when more is consumed in the diet. In all of these cases, the need for water increases in order to produce more urine to excrete the extra wastes.

The amount of water lost in the feces is usually small, only about 100 to 200 ml per day (less than a cup). This is remarkable because every day about 9 liters of fluid enter the gastrointestinal tract via food, water, and gastrointestinal secretions. Under normal

---

FACT BOX 6.1

Death by Dehydration

When you have diarrhea, you lose a lot of water. Too much water loss is fatal. Every year, about 4 billion cases of diarrhea occur, causing 2.2 million deaths, mostly among children under the age of five. This is equivalent to one child dying every 15 seconds. These diarrhea-related deaths represent approximately 15% of all child deaths under the age of five in developing countries. The diarrhea is caused by bacterial and viral infections. One of these infections, called cholera, can cause a person to lose 2 to 3 gallons of fluid a day. Survival often depends on the administration of intravenous fluids to replace these staggering losses. Improving water quality, sanitation, and hygiene in under-developed countries could significantly reduce diarrheal diseases and the number of deaths from dehydration.

conditions, more than 95% is reabsorbed before the feces are elimi-nated. However, in cases of severe diarrhea, large amounts of water can be lost through the gastrointestinal tract.

Water loss due to evaporation from the skin and respiratory tract takes place continuously. These losses are referred to as **insensible losses** because the individual is unaware that it is occurring. An inactive person at room temperature loses about 1,000 ml per day through insensible losses, but the amount varies depending on body size, environmental temperature and humidity, and physical activity. For example, more water is lost when the humidity is low, such as in the desert, than would be lost on a rainy day.

Water is also lost in sweat. The amount of water lost through sweat is extremely variable depending on environmental conditions (temperature, humidity, wind speed, radiant heat), clothing, exercise intensity, level of physical training, and acclimation to the environ-ment. Sweat rate increases as exercise intensity increases and as the environment becomes hotter and more humid. An individual doing light work at a temperature of about 84°F (29°C) will lose about 2 to 3 liters of sweat per day. Strenuous exercise in a hot environment can cause water losses in sweat to be as high as 2 to 4 liters in an hour.[12] Clothing that allows the evaporation of sweat will permit the body to be cooled and will decrease sweat losses (Figure 6.2).

Kidneys Regulate Water Excretion

The kidneys serve as a filtering system that regulates the amount of water and dissolved substances retained in the blood and excreted in the urine. As blood flows through the kidneys, water and small molecules are filtered out. Some of the water and molecules are reabsorbed into the blood and the rest are excreted in the urine. The amount of water and electrolytes that are reabsorbed depends on conditions in the body. There are two hormonal systems that regulate fluid balance.

One of these systems detects changes in the concentration of solutes in the blood. When the concentration of solutes in the blood is high, the pituitary gland secretes **antidiuretic hormone (ADH)**. This hormone signals the kidneys to reabsorb water, reducing the

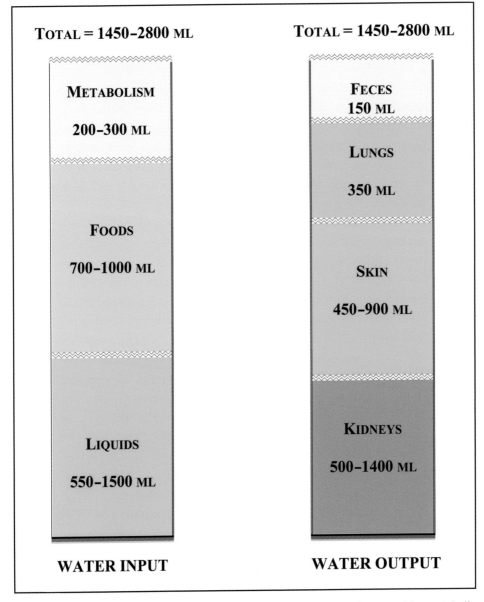

Figure 6.2 Water enters the body in liquids and foods, and some is created by metabolic processes. Water leaves the body in urine (kidneys), feces, through sweat and evaporation from the skin, and moisture in exhaled air (lungs). This figure illustrates the approximate amounts of water that come into the body from various sources and the approximate amounts lost in various ways in a person who is not sweating.

amount lost in the urine. This reabsorbed water is returned to the blood, decreasing the solute concentration to normal. When the solute concentration in the blood is low, ADH levels decrease, so less water is reabsorbed and more is excreted in the urine, allowing blood solute concentration to increase to normal.

The other system that regulates the amount of water in the body is activated by changes in blood pressure and relies on the ability of the kidneys to conserve the mineral sodium. Because water follows sodium by osmosis, changes in the amount of sodium retained or excreted result in changes in the amount of body water. Sodium is located primarily outside of cells where it is the primary determinant of extracellular fluid volume. When the concentration of sodium in the blood decreases, water moves out of the blood, causing a decrease in blood volume. A decrease in blood volume can cause a decrease in blood pressure. When blood pressure decreases, the kidneys release the enzyme **renin**, beginning a series of events that leads to the production of **angiotensin II** (Figure 6.3). Angiotensin II increases blood pressure both by causing the blood vessel walls to constrict and by stimulating the release of the hormone **aldosterone**, which acts on the kidneys to increase sodium reabsorption. Water follows the reabsorbed sodium, and is returned to the blood. As blood pressure returns to normal, it inhibits the release of renin and aldosterone so that blood pressure does not continue to rise.

DEHYDRATION: TOO LITTLE BODY WATER

When water loss exceeds water intake, dehydration results. Dehydration severe enough to cause clinical symptoms can occur more rapidly than any other nutrient deficiency. Likewise, health can be restored in a matter of minutes or hours when fluid is replaced.

Early symptoms of dehydration include headache, fatigue, loss of appetite, dry eyes and mouth, and concentrated urine, which is dark in color. Even mild dehydration—a body water loss of 1% to 2% of body weight—can impair physical and cognitive performance.[13] When 3% or more of body weight is lost as water, there can be

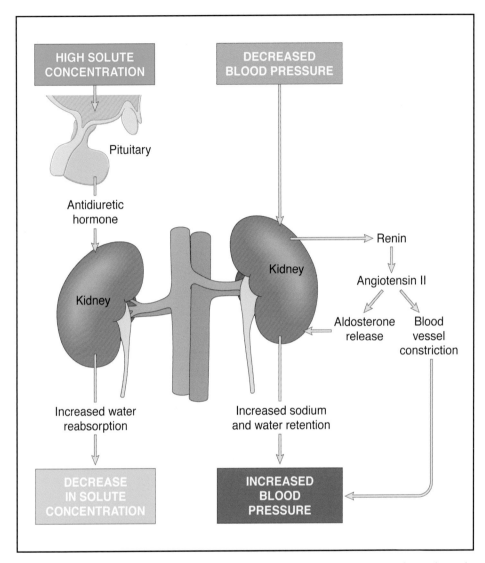

Figure 6.3 Fluid balance is regulated by antidiuretic hormone and the renin-angiotensin system, which triggers the release of the hormone aldosterone.

significant reductions in the amount of blood pumped by the heart. This reduces the ability to deliver oxygen and nutrients to cells and remove waste products. As blood volume decreases, it also reduces blood flow to the skin and sweat production,

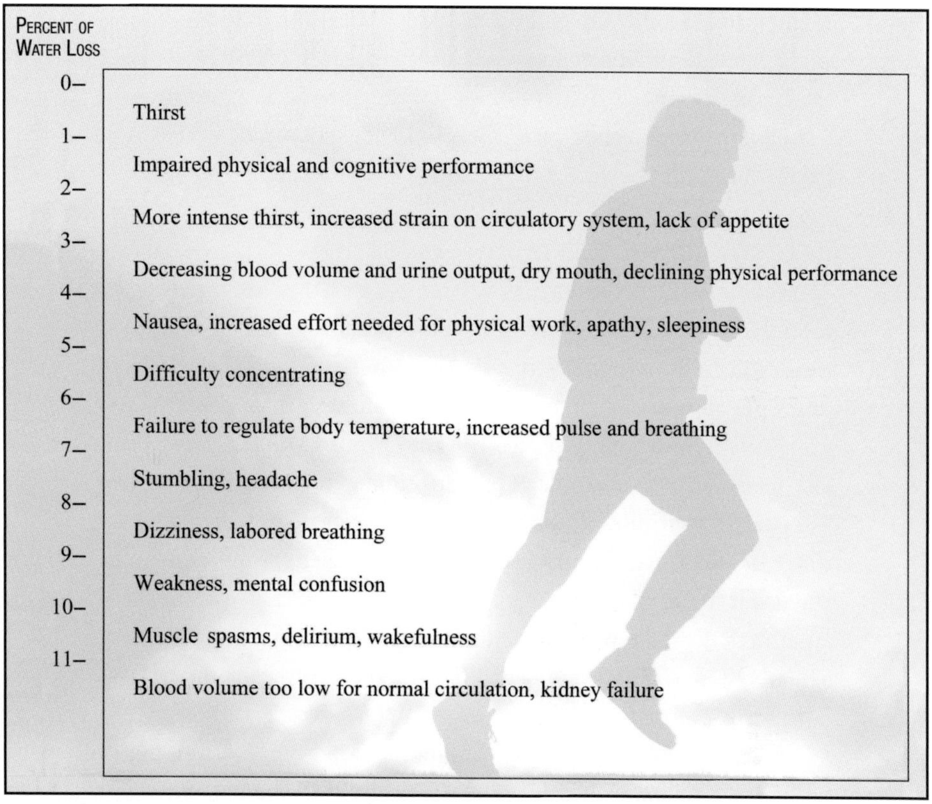

PERCENT OF
WATER LOSS

0–	
1–	Thirst
2–	Impaired physical and cognitive performance
3–	More intense thirst, increased strain on circulatory system, lack of appetite
4–	Decreasing blood volume and urine output, dry mouth, declining physical performance
5–	Nausea, increased effort needed for physical work, apathy, sleepiness
6–	Difficulty concentrating
7–	Failure to regulate body temperature, increased pulse and breathing
8–	Stumbling, headache
9–	Dizziness, labored breathing
10–	Weakness, mental confusion
11–	Muscle spasms, delirium, wakefulness
	Blood volume too low for normal circulation, kidney failure

Figure 6.4 As the amount of water loss increases, the effects of dehydration become more severe.

which limits the body's ability to sweat and cool itself. Body temperature then increases and, with it, the risk of various heat-related disorders. As water losses increase, a proportionately greater percentage of the water is lost from intracellular spaces. This water is needed to maintain metabolic functions. A loss of 5% of body water can cause nausea and difficulty concentrating. When water loss approaches 7%, confusion and disorientation may occur. A loss of about 10% to 20% can result in death (Figure 6.4).

The risk of dehydration is increased in infants and the elderly because their kidneys are inefficient at concentrating urine. Also, infants and debilitated elderly individuals cannot ask for liquids when they are thirsty. Athletes are at risk because of the large water losses that occur with strenuous exercise. Staying well hydrated is particularly important if you are exercising because a decrease in body water causes a decline in athletic performance.

CAN YOU DRINK TOO MUCH WATER?

Too much water, or water toxicity, can occur either because there is too much water in the body or because there is too little sodium, a condition called **hyponatremia**. This can occur as a result of illness, improper administration of intravenous fluids, or from drinking too much plain water when excessive amounts of sodium have been lost in sweat. For example, hyponatremia can occur if an athlete loses large amounts of water and salt in sweat, but drinks plain water to rehydrate. It is also possible to develop hyponatremia even when salt losses from sweating are not excessive. This can occur if an athlete drinks too much water, which dilutes the sodium in his or her system. It is the concentration of sodium that is important, not the absolute amount.

A low concentration of sodium in the blood causes a number of problems. Solutes in the blood help hold fluid in the blood vessels. As sodium concentration drops, fluid will leave the bloodstream by osmosis and accumulate in the tissues, causing swelling. Fluid accumulation in the lungs interferes with gas exchange and fluid

---

FACT BOX 6.2

Can Athletes Drink Enough?

During exercise, most people only drink enough to quench their thirst. That means they end their exercise session in a state of dehydration and must restore fluid balance during the post-exercise period. Even when endurance athletes consume fluids at regular intervals throughout exercise, they often cannot take in enough to compensate for losses in sweat and evaporation through the lungs and, as a result, they may suffer the effects of dehydration.

accumulation in the brain causes disorientation, seizure, coma, and death. The early symptoms of hyponatremia may be similar to dehydration: nausea, muscle cramps, disorientation, slurred speech, and confusion. Drinking water alone will make the problem worse and can result in seizure, coma, or death.

HOW MUCH WATER DO YOU NEED?

The recommendation for total water intake is about 2.7 liters per day for women and 3.7 liters per day for men. This does not all need to be consumed as water; other fluids such as juice and milk, as well as the water in foods, contribute to needs. In a typical diet, 30% of the water is consumed in fluids and 20% comes from foods. Although beverages that contain caffeine, such as coffee, tea, and caffeinated soda, cause water to be lost from the body, such beverages still contribute to maintaining water balance.

Three to 4 liters of fluid per day is sufficient under average conditions, but water needs can be increased by variations in activity, environment, and diet. Exercise increases water needs because it increases evaporative losses and sweating. Athletes can estimate water loss by weighing themselves before and after exercise. To restore fluid balance, about 3 cups (0.7 liters) of fluid should be consumed for every pound of weight lost. A dry environment also increases water losses because more moisture is lost to the environment from evaporation from the skin and lungs. Low-calorie diets can also increase water needs because extra urine is produced in order to excrete ketones produced by fat breakdown.

Water needs are higher at certain life stages. They are proportionately higher during infancy because the infant's kidneys cannot concentrate urine as efficiently as adult kidneys, so water loss is greater. Infants also lose proportionately more water through evaporation because their surface area is large relative to body weight. An intake of 3 cups per day for a six-month-old infant is recommended. Water needs are higher during pregnancy in order to allow for the increase in maternal blood volume, the production of amniotic fluid, and the needs of the fetus. During lactation, fluid needs are increased because the fluid secreted in milk, about 3 cups (0.7 liters) per day, must be restored by the mother's fluid intake.

CONNECTIONS

Water is an essential nutrient. In the body, it transports nutrients and other substances; provides structure and protection; is needed for numerous chemical reactions; and is extremely important in the regulation of body temperature. Water is distributed between intra-cellular and extracellular compartments and moves between these by osmosis. Water cannot be stored, so intake must equal output to maintain hydration. Water is consumed in beverages and food and

---

FACT BOX 6.3

Getting Enough Water Before, During, and After Exercise

Exercise increases water needs. Make sure you get enough of the right kinds of fluids to optimize your exercise by following these suggestions:

BEFORE EXERCISE

- Begin exercise well hydrated by consuming generous amounts of fluid in the 24 hours before exercise.
- Consume about 2 cups of fluid 2 hours before exercise.

DURING EXERCISE

- Consume at least 6 to 12 ounces of fluid every 15 to 20 minutes.
- For exercise lasting 60 minutes or less, water is adequate for fluid replacement.
- For exercise lasting longer than 60 minutes, a fluid containing carbohydrates and electrolytes may improve endurance and protect health.

AFTER EXERCISE

- Begin fluid replacement immediately after exercise.
- Consume 24 ounces of fluid for each pound of weight lost.

small amounts are produced by metabolism in the body. Water is excreted in the urine and feces and lost in sweat and through evaporation from the skin and lungs. Water balance is primarily regulated by the kidneys. If body water is low, antidiuretic hormone causes a reduction in urine output and other hormones cause the kidney to retain sodium, thereby increasing water retention. A reduction in body water can have dire consequences for health. Mild dehydration can result in headache, fatigue, loss of appetite, and concentrated dark-colored urine. More severe dehydration can interfere with the functioning of the circulatory system and the ability of the body to cool itself and can be fatal.

7

Vitamins

What comes to mind when you think of vitamins? Many of us think of energy, but vitamins don't provide you with energy. They do play a role in energy production because some are needed to regulate the reactions that form ATP from carbohydrates, fats, and proteins. In addition to this role, vitamins are involved in a multitude of other body processes, from bone formation to antioxidant protection.

SOME VITAMINS DISSOLVE IN WATER AND SOME DISSOLVE IN FAT

Vitamins are organic compounds that are essential in the diet in small amounts to promote and regulate body functions. When the diet is deficient in a particular vitamin, deficiency symptoms develop. These symptoms are relieved when the vitamin is added back to the diet. Vitamins are generally classified based on whether they dissolve in water or fat because this property affects how vitamins are absorbed, transported, excreted, and stored in the body. The **water-soluble vitamins** include the B vitamins (thiamin, riboflavin, niacin, biotin, pantothenic acid, vitamin B_6, folate, and vitamin B_{12}) and vitamin C. The **fat-soluble vitamins** include vitamins A, D, E, and K. Fat-soluble vitamins are best absorbed when they are consumed with other fats in the diet and, once inside the body, they are transported with fat. Water-soluble vitamins do not need fat for absorption but may need energy-requiring transport systems or special molecules that bind them in the gastrointestinal tract to be absorbed. Some must also be attached to specific proteins to be transported in the blood. With the exception of vitamin B_{12}, water-soluble vitamins consumed in excess of needs are excreted in the urine. Fat-soluble vitamins, on the other hand, are not excreted in the urine but rather are stored in the liver and fatty tissues. Therefore, it takes longer to develop a deficiency of vitamin B_{12} and fat-soluble vitamins when they are no longer included in the diet.

HOW MUCH DO WE NEED?

The amount of each vitamin a person needs to remain healthy varies depending on his or her age, gender, size, and life stage as well as health status. DRIs have established population recommendations for the amounts of each vitamin needed to prevent deficiency and promote health (Table 7.1). For some vitamins, a Tolerable Upper Intake Level (UL) has also been established; intakes above these levels increase the risk of toxicity (see Appendix B).

THIAMIN

In East Asian countries, the thiamin deficiency disease **beriberi** has been known for over 1,000 years. It became more widespread in the 1800s when the practice of polishing off the bran layer of brown rice to create polished white rice became popular. Although this created a more uniform product, it also removed the vitamin-rich portion of the grain and created a dietary deficiency of thiamin. Today, the incidence of beriberi in Asia is markedly decreased, partly because an improved standard of living has allowed a more varied diet and partly because of the introduction and gradual acceptance of **enriched** rice and other forms of rice that contain higher concentrations of thiamin.

Table 7.1 Recommended Vitamin Intakes

VITAMIN	RECOMMENDED INTAKE FOR ADULTS
Thiamin	1.1–1.2 mg
Riboflavin	1.1–1.3 mg
Niacin	14–16 mg NE
Biotin	30 μg
Pantothenic acid	5 mg
Vitamin B$_6$	1.3–1.7 mg
Folate	400 μg DFE
Vitamin B$_{12}$	2.4 μg
Vitamin C	75–90 mg
Vitamin A	700–900 μg
Vitamin D	5–15 μg
Vitamin E	15 mg
Vitamin K	90–120 μg
NE: Niacin Equivalents	DFE: Dietary Folate Equivalents

Beriberi affects the nervous and cardiovascular systems. The earliest symptoms of depression and weakness occur after only about ten days on a thiamin-free diet. Other neurological symptoms include poor coordination, tingling, and paralysis. In North America today, thiamin deficiency is rare but it does occur in alcoholics partly because alcohol decreases thiamin absorption. Thiamin-deficient alcoholics may develop a neurological condition known as the Wernicke-Korsakoff syndrome, characterized by mental confusion, psychosis, memory disturbances, and coma.

Thiamin is a B vitamin needed as a **coenzyme** for some of the important energy-yielding reactions in the body. Coenzymes are nonprotein organic molecules that act as enzyme helpers in metabolic reactions. The active coenzyme form of thiamin, thiamin pyrophosphate, is needed in reactions in which carbon dioxide is lost from larger molecules. This includes two reactions needed for the production of energy from glucose. Since the brain and nervous tissue rely on glucose for energy, some the symptoms of beriberi may be related to the inability to use glucose completely. Symptoms such as poor coordination, tingling, and paralysis may also be related to thiamin's role in the synthesis of acetylcholine, which is needed to transmit nerve signals. Thiamin is also needed for the metabolism of other sugars and certain amino acids and the synthesis of ribose, a sugar that is part of the structure of RNA (ribonucleic acid).

Good sources of thiamin in the diet include pork, whole grains, legumes, nuts, seeds, and organ meats (liver, kidney, heart). It is one of the vitamins added to enriched grain products such as breads and pasta. Some foods such as raw shellfish and freshwater fish, tea, coffee, betel nuts, blueberries, and red cabbage contain substances that destroy thiamin during storage, preparation, or passage through the gastrointestinal tract. Because these antithiamin factors make thiamin unavailable to the body, habitual consumption of these foods increases the risk of thiamin deficiency. No toxicity has been reported when excess thiamin is consumed from either food or supplements.

FACT BOX 7.1

Beriberi: The Chicken Connection

Beriberi was a major problem in colonial Asia in the 19th century. It was affecting so many soldiers that in 1886, the Dutch government sent a commission to its colony in Java to determine the cause. After several failed attempts to duplicate the disease in chickens, the birds suddenly developed beriberi-like symptoms and many died. Then, just as quickly, the surviving chickens recovered. An observant young medical officer named Christian Eijkman noted that the epidemic occurred when a shipment of brown rice failed to arrive and the chickens were given white rice instead. The epidemic subsided when the superintendent found out that chickens were being fed expensive white rice and switched them back to brown rice. The reason brown rice prevented beriberi would not be revealed until 1912 when Casamir Funk isolated a substance from rice husks that prevented beriberi and coined the term *vitamine.*

RIBOFLAVIN

Years ago, the milkman used to deliver glass bottles of milk to people's houses. Did you ever wonder why milk doesn't come in clear glass bottles any more? Well, in addition to the fact that the bottles are breakable and hard to clean, the B vitamin riboflavin is sensitive to light. Milk is one of the best sources of riboflavin in the North American diet, and, if it is in a container that exposes it to light, much of the riboflavin will be destroyed. The most riboflavin-friendly milk containers are opaque to protect the thiamin from light. Other good dietary sources of riboflavin include meat, asparagus, broccoli, mushrooms, leafy green vegetables, and whole and enriched grains.

Riboflavin is needed to produce energy from carbohydrate, fat, and protein. It has two active coenzyme forms: flavin adenine dinucleotide (FAD) and flavin mononucleotide (FMN). FAD functions in the citric acid cycle and both FAD and FMN function as electron carriers in the electron transport chain. Riboflavin is also needed to convert a number of other vitamins, including folate, niacin, vitamin B_6, and vitamin K, into their active forms.

Riboflavin deficiency, called **ariboflavinosis**, is uncommon and usually occurs in conjunction with deficiencies of other B vitamins. Symptoms include inflammation of the eyes, lips, mouth, and tongue; scaly, greasy skin eruptions; cracking of the tissue at the corners of the mouth; and confusion. No adverse effects have been reported from overconsumption of riboflavin from foods or supplements.

NIACIN

In the early 1900s, the niacin deficiency disease **pellagra** was epidemic in the southeastern United States. Pellagra was prevalent because the local diet among the poor consisted of cornmeal, molasses, and fatback or salt pork—all poor sources of niacin. Pellagra causes symptoms that can be remembered as the three Ds: dermatitis, diarrhea, and dementia. If untreated, a fourth "D" results—death. Pellagra remained a problem in the United States until World War II (1939–1945), when economic changes led to a better diet and a federally sponsored enrichment program added niacin, thiamin, and riboflavin to grains. Today, pellagra has been virtually eliminated in the United States but remains common in India and parts of China and Africa.

Niacin is a B vitamin that functions in energy production and in reactions that synthesize fatty acids and cholesterol. There are two forms of niacin: nicotinic acid and nicotinamide. Both can be used to make the active coenzyme forms nicotinamide adenine dinucleotide (NAD) and nicotinamide adenine dinucleotide phosphate (NADP). NAD is needed in the citric acid cycle and NADP is needed to synthesize fatty acids and cholesterol.

Niacin is found primarily in meat and fish, but legumes, mushrooms, wheat bran, asparagus, peanuts, and whole and enriched grains are also good sources. Niacin can be synthesized in

---

FACT BOX 7.2

The Mystery of Pellagra

In the early 1900s, psychiatric hospitals in the southern United States were filled with patients with the disease pellagra. At that time, no one knew what caused it. Some felt it was due to an infection or a toxin. It was the observations and experiments of Dr. Joseph Goldberger, who was sent by the Public Health Service to investigate the pellagra epidemic, which finally unraveled the mystery. He observed that individuals in institutions such as hospitals, orphanages, and prisons suffered from pellagra, but the staff did not. If pellagra were an infectious disease, both populations would be equally affected. He hypothesized that pellagra was due to a deficiency in the diet. To test his hypothesis, nutritious foods such as fresh meats, milk, and eggs were added to the diet of children in orphanages. The symptoms of pellagra disappeared, supporting the hypothesis that pellagra is due to a deficiency of something in the diet. In another experiment, he was able to induce pellagra in healthy prison inmates by feeding them an unhealthy diet. These experiments and others supported the hypothesis that pellagra is caused by a dietary deficiency. The vitamin niacin was not identified until 1937. The discovery of the relationship between nutrition and pellagra, a disease now known to be caused by a niacin deficiency, is an example of how scientific investigations have led to nutrition discoveries.

the body from the essential amino acid tryptophan. In a diet that is high in protein but low in niacin, much of the needed niacin can be made from tryptophan. However, when available tryptophan is needed to synthesize body proteins, it is not used to synthesize niacin.

High niacin intakes from supplements can cause toxicity symptoms including flushing, tingling in the hands and feet, a red skin rash, nausea, vomiting, diarrhea, high blood sugar levels, abnormalities in liver function, and blurred vision. In those who can tolerate it, doses of 50 mg per day or greater of nicotinic acid have been shown to decrease blood levels of LDL cholesterol and triglycerides and increase HDL cholesterol. This amount is also associated with a reduction in second heart attacks in individuals with cardiovascular disease.[14]

BIOTIN

Biotin is a B vitamin that is important in the citric acid cycle and is needed for the synthesis of glucose and the metabolism of fatty acids and amino acids. Biotin acts as a coenzyme for a group of enzymes that add the acid group COOH to molecules. Sources of biotin in the diet include liver, egg yolks, yogurt, and nuts. Raw egg whites contain a protein called avidin that binds biotin, making it unavailable to the body. Cooking eggs denatures avidin so that it cannot bind biotin. Biotin deficiency is uncommon but has been seen in people with protein energy malnutrition and those fed intravenous solutions of nutrients that are lacking biotin.

PANTOTHENIC ACID

Pantothenic acid is part of the structure of coenzyme A (CoA). Co-enzyme A is needed to make acetyl CoA, a molecule formed during the breakdown of carbohydrates, fatty acids, and amino acids. Pantothenic acid is also part of a protein needed for the synthesis of cholesterol and fatty acids. It is particularly abundant in meat, eggs, whole grains, and legumes and is found in lesser amounts in milk, vegetables, and fruits. The wide distribution of pantothenic acid in foods makes human deficiency rare; it may occur as a result of malnutrition or chronic alcoholism when many B vitamins are deficient.

VITAMIN B$_6$

The chemical term for vitamin B$_6$ is **pyridoxine**, but you may not recognize this name because this vitamin is one of only two B vitamins that we still commonly refer to by a number (vitamin B$_{12}$ is the other). It is important in protein and amino acid metabolism; without vitamin B$_6$, the nonessential amino acids cannot be made in the body. Vitamin B$_6$ has three forms—pyridoxal, pyridoxine, and pyridoxamine. These can be converted into the active coenzyme form, pyridoxal phosphate, which is needed for the activity of more than 100 enzymes involved in the metabolism of carbohydrates, fat, and protein. Pyridoxine functions in the immune system and the synthesis of hemoglobin, certain neurotransmitters, and lipids that are part of the myelin coating on nerves. It is also needed for the metabolism of the carbohydrate storage molecule glycogen and for the synthesis of niacin from tryptophan.

Vitamin B$_6$ is found in chicken, fish, pork, and organ meats as well as whole grains, soybeans, sunflower seeds, and some fruits and vegetables such as bananas, broccoli, and spinach.

Vitamin B$_6$ status in the body can be affected by a number of drugs, including alcohol and oral contraceptives. Symptoms of vitamin B$_6$ deficiency include depression, headaches, confusion, numbness and tingling in the extremities, and seizures; these may be related to the role of vitamin B$_6$ in neurotransmitter synthesis and myelin formation. Anemia may occur due to B$_6$ deficiency because of the vitamin's role in hemoglobin synthesis.

A deficiency of vitamin B$_6$ may also be involved in the development of heart disease. When vitamin B$_6$ is not available, an amino acid called homocysteine accumulates in the blood. High levels of homocystiene increase the risk for cardiovascular disease (Figure 7.1). Vitamin B$_{12}$ and folate are also needed to prevent homocysteine accumulation.

Low-dose supplements may be beneficial in reducing the anxiety, irritability, and depression associated with premenstrual syndrome (PMS).[15] Vitamin B$_6$ supplements have been found to improve immune function in older adults, but since the elderly frequently have low intakes of vitamin B$_6$, it is unclear whether the beneficial

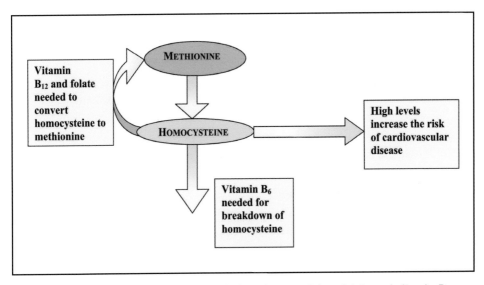

Figure 7.1 Vitamin B$_6$ is needed to break down homocysteine; folate and vitamin B$_{12}$ are needed to convert homocysteine back to methionine. If any of these vitamins is deficient, homocysteine levels in the body will increase, raising the risk of heart disease.

effects of supplements are due to an improvement in vitamin B$_6$ status or immune system stimulation.

Although supplements may be important for some people, be aware that vitamin B$_6$ is toxic. Excessive intakes of vitamin B$_6$ can cause irreversible nerve damage that affects the ability to walk and causes numbness in the extremities. Intakes greater than 100 mg per day are not recommended.

FOLATE OR FOLIC ACID

Low intakes of folate have been associated with birth defects that affect the brain and spinal cord called neural tube defects. The connection between folate intake and neural tube defects is so strong that the U.S. government requires folic acid to be added to breads, cereals, and other grain products. Folic acid is a stable form of folate that is used in fortified foods and supplements. Between 1998, when grain products were first fortified with folic acid, and 2001, the incidence of neural tube defects decreased by 19%.[16]

In the body, the B vitamin folate is needed for the synthesis of DNA and the metabolism of some amino acids. Because a cell must synthesize DNA in order to divide, folate is particularly important when cells are dividing rapidly. A deficiency causes a form of anemia called macrocytic or megaloblastic anemia, which is characterized by large red blood cells. This occurs because the red blood cells cannot duplicate their DNA; they therefore grow bigger but cannot divide. In addition to anemia, folate deficiency causes poor growth, abnormalities in nerve development and function, diarrhea, and inflammation of the tongue.

Low intakes of folate are associated with an increased risk of heart disease, cancer, and birth defects. The connection between low intakes of folate and heart disease is the amino acid homocysteine. When folate intake is low, homocysteine can build up in the blood, increasing the risk of heart disease. Low folate intake also increases the risk of colon cancer and possibly cancers of the uterus, cervix, lung, stomach, and esophagus. The cancer risk associated with a low folate diet is greatly increased by alcohol consumption. A low intake of folate in early pregnancy increases the risk of neural tube defects. Although low folate is not the only cause, supplemental folic acid, taken before and during early pregnancy, has been associated with a reduced incidence of these birth defects. Because of this, it is recommended that women who are capable of becoming pregnant consume folic acid from fortified foods or supplements in addition to the folate in a balanced diet. Dietary sources of folate include enriched grains, liver, asparagus, corn, snap beans, mustard greens, broccoli, oranges, legumes, and some nuts.

An excessive intake of folate is a concern because it can mask the symptoms of vitamin B_{12} deficiency and therefore may delay treatment until damage becomes permanent.

VITAMIN B_{12}

Vitamin B_{12}, or **cobalamin**, is a B vitamin that is found only in animal products. Foods like beef, chicken, and fish are excellent dietary sources but plant foods do not provide this vitamin unless they have been contaminated with other sources of B_{12}, or have been fortified.

Vitamin B_{12} is necessary for the maintenance of myelin, which insulates nerves and is necessary for nerve transmission. One B_{12}-dependent reaction rearranges carbon atoms so that fatty acids can be used to generate energy. A second reaction synthesizes the amino acid methionine from homocysteine. This reaction also regenerates the active coenzyme form of folate, which is needed for DNA synthesis. Because of the need for vitamin B_{12} in folate metabolism, a deficiency of vitamin B_{12} can cause a folate deficiency and excesses of folate can mask a vitamin B_{12} deficiency.

Because vitamin B_{12} is needed in folate metabolism, some of the deficiency symptoms are the same for these two vitamins—elevated blood homocysteine levels and macrocytic anemia. Because vitamin B_{12} is needed to maintain the myelin sheath that coats the nerves, B_{12} deficiency also causes neurological symptoms including tingling and numbness, abnormalities in gait, memory loss, and disorientation.

Vitamin B_{12} in food is bound to protein. In order to be absorbed, it must be released by protein-digesting enzymes and bound to **intrinsic factor**, a protein secreted by the stomach. Only a very small amount of vitamin B_{12} can be absorbed without intrinsic factor.

Vitamin B_{12} deficiency takes a long time to develop even if the diet is deficient because the vitamin is efficiently recycled. It is secreted into bile, and when the bile enters the gastrointestinal tract, most of the B_{12} is reabsorbed. Deficiencies occur in individuals who consume no animal products and in those with pernicious anemia, an autoimmune disease in which the cells that produce intrinsic factor are destroyed. Individuals with an inflammation of the stomach lining called atrophic gastritis are also at risk for deficiency. Atrophic gastritis causes a reduction in stomach acid, which reduces the absorption of vitamin B_{12} that is bound to proteins in food. This condition occurs in 10% to 30% of individuals over 50 years of age. Because it is so common, it is recommended that individuals over the age of 50 meet their RDA for vitamin B_{12} by consuming fortified foods or by taking a vitamin B_{12}-containing supplement. The vitamin B_{12} in fortified foods and supplements is not bound to proteins so it is absorbed even when stomach acid is low.

VITAMIN C

Throughout history, the vitamin C deficiency disease **scurvy** has been the downfall of armies, navies, and explorers. The reason this vitamin was a particular problem is that it is found in fresh fruits and vegetables—foods that spoil quickly and do not transport well on long voyages. In the 17th century, Sir Richard Hawkins observed that scurvy could be cured by consuming citrus fruit. Unfortunately, this did not become common practice until about 150 years later when it became mandatory for British sailors to include lime or lemon juice in their rations, earning them the name "limeys."

Vitamin C, also known as **ascorbate** or **ascorbic acid**, is a water-soluble vitamin needed for the synthesis and maintenance of **collagen**, the predominant protein in connective tissue. Without sufficient vitamin C, collagen cannot be synthesized or maintained. This causes the symptoms of scurvy, which include poor wound healing, weakened blood vessels, bone fractures, bleeding gums, and loose teeth.

Vitamin C is also needed for the synthesis of some neurotransmitters and hormones, bile acids, and carnitine, which is needed to break down fatty acids. Vitamin C also acts as an antioxidant, a substance that protects against damage from reactive oxygen molecules such as free radicals. These reactive molecules damage DNA, proteins, carbohydrates, and unsaturated fatty acids by stealing their electrons. Antioxidants protect the body by destroying reactive oxygen molecules before they can do damage. Some antioxidants are produced in the body; others, including vitamin C, vitamin E, and the mineral selenium, are dietary constituents. The antioxidant properties of vitamin C also allow it to regenerate the active antioxidant form of vitamin E and enhance iron absorption by keeping iron in its more readily absorbed form.

The best-known source of vitamin C is citrus fruits such as oranges, lemons, and limes. Other good sources include strawberries, cantaloupe, tomatoes, peppers, potatoes, leafy green vegetables, and vegetables in the cabbage family, such as broccoli, cauliflower, bok choy, and brussels sprouts.

In the United States today, scurvy is rare, but vitamin C is the most commonly consumed vitamin supplement. One-third of the population of the United States takes supplements of vitamin C in the hope that it will prevent or reduce cold symptoms. Scientific studies have shown that vitamin C does not reduce the incidence of colds but can reduce the duration and severity of cold symptoms.[17]

Vitamin C is relatively nontoxic, but intakes of more than 1 gram can cause diarrhea, nausea, and abdominal cramps. When vitamin C tablets are chewed, its acidic nature can cause tooth enamel to dissolve. High intakes of vitamin C can cause kidney stones in people prone to stone formation and worsen symptoms in those with sickle-cell anemia.

VITAMIN A

Did anyone ever tell you to eat your carrots because they will help you see in the dark? Well, they were right. Carrots are a good source of **beta-carotene** (β-carotene), which can be turned into vitamin A in your body. Vitamin A is needed for vision; one of the first signs of a deficiency is trouble adapting to dim light at night, called night blindness.

Vitamin A is a fat-soluble vitamin that comes in several different forms. **Retinoids** are preformed vitamin A. They are important for vision and **cell differentiation**, which is the process whereby immature cells change in structure and function to form mature specialized cells. Retinoids include retinal, retinol, and retinoic acid. Carotenoids, such as β-carotene, are vitamin A precursors that can be converted to retinoids in the body.

Because retinoids and carotenoids are fat soluble, they are absorbed along with dietary fat. In the small intestine, they, along with other fat-soluble food components, combine with bile acids to form micelles, which facilitate their absorption.[19] Retinoids are absorbed more efficiently than carotenoids. From the intestine, retinoids and carotenoids are transported along with dietary fat in lipoproteins and delivered to body cells. Retinoids are stored in the liver. To move from liver stores to the tissues, preformed vitamin A must be bound to retinol-binding protein.

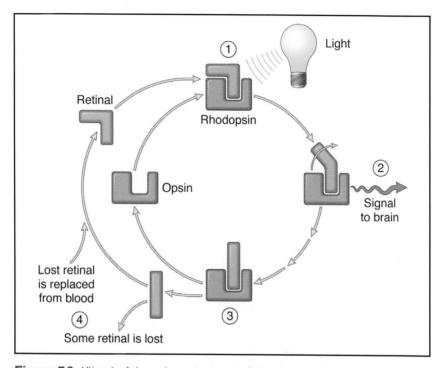

Figure 7.2 Vitamin A is an important part of the visual cycle. In the eye, retinal combines with opsin to form rhodopsin (1). When light strikes rhodopsin, retinal changes shape, causing a nerve signal to be sent to the brain (2) and retinal to separate from opsin (3). Some of this retinol is lost and must be replaced from retinoids in the blood (4).

The different forms of vitamin A have different functions. The retinal form is important in the visual cycle. In this cycle, retinal combines with the protein opsin to form the visual pigment **rhodopsin** (Figure 7.2). When stimulated by light, the retinal in rhodopsin is changed from a curved molecule into a straight one. This change causes retinal to separate from opsin and sends a nerve signal to the brain. After the light stimulus has passed, the retinal can be converted back to its curved form and rhodopsin can be regenerated. Each time this cycle occurs, some retinal is lost and must be replaced by vitamin A from the blood. If vitamin A is deficient, this cannot be replaced and night blindness occurs.

The retinoic acid form of vitamin A can be made from retinol or retinal. It affects cell differentiation by affecting gene expression. In other words, retinoic acid affects which genes are turned on and which are turned off. In this way, it determines which proteins a cell will produce. In epithelial tissues, which line and cover surfaces, vitamin A is needed for the differentiation of cells into mucus-secreting cells. Without vitamin A, the cells do not differentiate properly and, instead of becoming mucus-secreting cells, they become cells that produce **keratin**, the hard protein that makes up hair and fingernails. When this occurs, the tissue becomes hard and dry and is at greater risk of infection. The eye is particularly susceptible to damage because the mucus secretions normally provide lubrication, wash away dirt, and destroy bacteria. Lack of mucus and the buildup of keratin leave the eye dry and open to infection. **Xerophthalmia** is a spectrum of eye conditions resulting from vitamin A deficiency. If not treated early, it can result in permanent blindness.

Vitamin A is important in reproduction because it is involved in directing cells to form each of the different tissues needed for a complete organism.[18] It is important in the immune system because it is needed for the differentiation of cells into the various types of immune cells. When vitamin A is deficient, immune function is impaired and the risk of illness and infection due to defective epithelial tissue barriers is increased.

Much of the β-carotene from the diet is converted into retinoids; however, some unconverted carotenoids also reach the blood and tissues, where they may function as antioxidants.

Vitamin A in the diet comes from both animal and plant sources. Retinoids are found in animal foods such as liver, fish, egg yolks, and dairy products. Margarine and nonfat and reduced-fat milk are fortified with retinoids because they are often consumed in place of butter and whole milk, which are good sources of this vitamin. Plant foods contain carotenoids. β-carotene is plentiful in carrots, squash, and other red and yellow vegetables and fruits as well as in leafy greens where the yellow-orange pigment is masked by green color of chlorophyll. Other carotenoids that can be converted into vitamin A include alpha-carotene, found in leafy green vegetables, carrots, and squash, and beta-cryptoxanthin found in corn, green peppers, and lemons. Lycopene, lutein, and zeaxanthin are carotenoids that cannot be converted into vitamin A.

Although uncommon in developed countries, vitamin A deficiency is a major public health problem in the developing world, particularly for children.[19] Children deficient in vitamin A are anemic, grow poorly, and are at increased risk for infections. It is estimated that 3 to 10 million children worldwide have xerophthalmia and 250,000 to 500,000 go blind annually due to vitamin A deficiency. A very low-fat diet, providing less than 10 grams per day, can cause a vitamin A deficiency because vitamin A cannot be absorbed from the diet without adequate fat. Protein deficiency can also precipitate vitamin A deficiency because protein is needed to transport the vitamin from stores in the liver.

Consumption of too much preformed vitamin A can be deadly. Common foods do not contain enough vitamin A to be a problem, but supplements of preformed vitamin A have the potential to deliver a toxic dose. Chronic toxicity occurs when preformed vitamin A doses as low as ten times the RDA are consumed for a period of months to years. Birth defects and bone loss are also associated with high dietary intakes of preformed vitamin A.[20] Carotenoids are not toxic, but a high intake can cause your skin to turn orange. To reduce the risk of toxicity, most supplements provide vitamin A as carotenoids.

FACT BOX 7.3

Pass on the Polar Bear Liver

In general, it is not possible to consume a toxic amount of a vitamin from a natural food. An exception is polar bear liver. In 1857, arctic explorers who consumed polar bear liver developed toxicity symptoms that included drowsiness, irritability, headache, and vomiting, with subsequent peeling of the skin. Why is polar bear liver so high in vitamin A? Vitamin A is stored in the liver and polar bears eat fish, seals, and walruses, all of which have enormous amounts of vitamin A stored in their livers. So, get your vitamin A by eating plenty of yellow-orange vegetables and fruits, and pass on the polar bear liver.

VITAMIN D

Vitamin D is a fat-soluble vitamin needed for healthy bones. It is known as the sunshine vitamin because it can be made in our skin when skin is exposed to sunlight. It is only essential in the diet when exposure to sunlight is limited or when the body's ability to make it is reduced. Lack of sunshine is the reason vitamin D deficiency was common in Europe during the Industrial Revolution. At this time, people moved from rural villages to big cities to work indoors in factories. Even when they were outside, smog and tall buildings blocked the sunlight. Today, vitamin D deficiency can still be a problem for inner-city children.

Vitamin D is also found in the diet in egg yolks, liver, and fatty fish such as salmon. These natural food sources of vitamin D contain vitamin D_3, or **cholecalciferol**, the form of vitamin D that is made in the skin. Foods that are fortified with vitamin D, such as milk and margarine, may contain either vitamin D_3 or D_2, another active form of the vitamin.

Vitamin D is needed for calcium absorption and to maintain the proper ratio of calcium and phosphorus in the blood. Whether made in the skin or consumed in the diet, in order to function, vitamin D must be converted to its active form. This involves the addition of 2 hydroxyl (OH) groups to its chemical structure. The first -OH is added by the liver and the second by the kidney. The activation of vitamin D occurs in response to **parathyroid hormone (PTH)**, which is released when blood calcium levels drop too low. At the intestine, active vitamin D turns on the synthesis of calcium transport proteins, which increase the absorption of calcium. At the bone, active vitamin D causes cells to differentiate into cells that break down bone. The breakdown of bone releases calcium and phosphorus into the blood. Vitamin D also acts with PTH to increase the amount of calcium retained by the kidneys.

When vitamin D is deficient, calcium absorption is reduced. Without sufficient calcium, bones are weakened. In children, vitamin D deficiency is called **rickets**. Rickets is characterized by narrow rib cages known as pigeon breasts and legs that bow because they are unable to support body weight (Figure 7.3). The fortification of

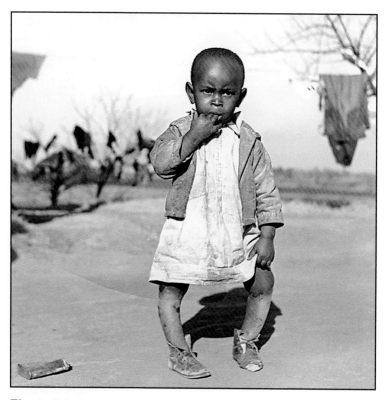

Figure 7.3 Bowed legs are characteristic of the vitamin D-deficiency disease rickets.

milk with vitamin D has helped to greatly reduce rickets in most developed countries but the incidence may be increasing due to lack of sun exposure and reduced consumption of milk. Dark-skinned children are more likely to be deficient because they require more time in the sun for enough vitamin D to be synthesized. In adults, vitamin D deficiency is called **osteomalacia**. It is characterized by a reduction in the mineral content of bone, leading to increased bone fractures. Osteomalacia is common in adults with kidney failure because the activation of vitamin D is reduced. Older adults are at increased risk because they generally spend less time in the sun and vitamin D production in the skin decreases with age. Another factor that may affect vitamin D status is the use of sunscreens. They block the ultraviolet light that is needed to produce vitamin D. However, most people spend enough time outside without sunscreen to meet their vitamin D needs. Those with dark skin pigmentation and those who live in northern climates may need to rely on dietary sources of the vitamin.

Vitamin D toxicity is rare. The synthesis of vitamin D in the skin is regulated and unfortified foods do not contain toxic amounts. Supplements containing vitamin D do pose a risk. Consuming 50 micrograms or more may cause symptoms that include high blood and urine calcium concentrations, deposition of calcium in the blood vessels and kidneys, and cardiovascular damage.

VITAMIN E

Vitamin E is a fat-soluble vitamin that was first recognized because it was necessary for fertility in laboratory rats. The chemical name for vitamin E is **tocopherol**, which is from the Greek *tos*, meaning "childbirth," and *phero*, "to bring forth."

Vitamin E functions as an antioxidant that neutralizes reactive oxygen compounds before they damage unsaturated fatty acids in cell membranes. After vitamin E is used to eliminate free radicals, its antioxidant function can be restored by vitamin C. Vitamin E is important in maintaining the integrity of red blood cells, cells in nervous tissue, and cells of the immune system. Vitamin E can also defend cells from damage caused by heavy metals, such as lead and mercury, and toxins, such as carbon tetrachloride, benzene, and a variety of drugs and environmental pollutants.

Vitamin E may help reduce the risk of heart disease in a number of ways. As an antioxidant, it may prevent the oxidation of LDL cholesterol, which is an early step in the development of atherosclerosis. It may also decrease the activity of enzymes involved in the formation of plaque in the arteries and it may increase the synthesis of enzymes needed for the production of eicosanoids, hormone-like molecules that help regulate blood pressure, blood clot formation, and immune function.[21] Although vitamin E supplements are often taken to reduce the risk of heart disease, the evidence for the benefit of supplements in protecting against heart disease is inconsistent.

There are several forms of vitamin E that occur naturally in food, but only **alpha-tocopherol (α-tocopherol)** can meet vitamin E requirements in humans. Synthetic α-tocopherol, found in dietary supplements and fortified foods, provides only half of the biological activity of natural α-tocopherol. Dietary sources of vitamin E include nuts and peanuts; plant oils such as soybean, corn, and sunflower oils; leafy green vegetables; wheat germ; and fortified breakfast cereals.

Vitamin E deficiency is rare because it is plentiful in the food supply and is stored in many of the body's tissues. A deficiency can cause changes in cell membranes; red blood cells and nerve tissue are particularly susceptible. Vitamin E is relatively nontoxic but supplements containing more than 1,000 mg/day can interfere with the activity of vitamin K.

VITAMIN K

Without vitamin K, a small scratch could cause you to bleed to death. This is because vitamin K is essential for blood clotting. When it is absent, even a small scratch could be fatal. This is how rat poison kills rodents. The main ingredient is a compound that inhibits vitamin K. When the rats eat it, their blood fails to clot and they bleed to death.

Some of the vitamin K we need is produced by bacteria that live in our intestines, but some must also come from the diet. **Phylloquinone** is the form of vitamin K found in plants. The best sources are leafy green vegetables such as spinach, broccoli, brussels sprouts, kale, and turnip greens. Vegetable oils including soybean, cottonseed, canola, and olive oil also provide vitamin K. **Menaquinones** are found in animal foods and dietary supplements; liver and fish oils are the best sources. Meats, milk, and eggs provide little of this vitamin. Menaquinones are the form synthesized by bacteria in the human intestine.

The major symptom of vitamin K deficiency is abnormal blood clotting. Deficiency is very rare in the healthy adult population, but it may result from fat malabsorption syndromes or the long-term use of antibiotics, which kill the bacteria in the gastrointestinal tract that are a source of the vitamin. Deficiency is a problem in newborns because little is transferred to the baby from the mother, breast milk is a poor source, and newborns have no bacteria in their gut to synthesize it. To ensure normal blood clotting, infants are typically given a vitamin K injection within 6 hours of birth.

The inability to form blood clots due to vitamin K deficiency or medications that interfere with vitamin K activity can cause death from excess blood loss. Blood thinning medications, such as coumadin, are routinely prescribed to prevent blood clots that cause heart attacks and strokes. Individuals taking these medications may need to avoid supplements containing vitamin K because it may reduce the effectiveness of the medication.

CONNECTIONS

Vitamins are organic compounds that are essential in the diet in small amounts to promote and regulate body functions. The

---

FACT BOX 7.4

Cows, Clover, and Coagulation

When President Dwight Eisenhower had a heart attack in 1955, his recovery was aided by an anticoagulant drug called sodium warfarin. Warfarin prevents blood from clotting by interfering with the action of vitamin K. It is still used today to prevent fatal blood clots in millions of people. The discovery of warfarin had its beginnings in the 1930s when cows across the midwestern prairies were bleeding to death from what was called hemorrhagic sweet clover disease. The wheels of science were set in motion on a snowy night in 1933 when a farmer delivered a bale of moldy clover hay, a pail of unclotted blood, and a dead cow to the laboratory of Dr. Carl Link at the University of Wisconsin. Link and his colleagues isolated the anticoagulant dicoumarol from the moldy clover. It was formed by the action of mold on a compound normally present in the clover, and when the cows consumed the moldy clover, their blood failed to clot. Dicoumarol was the first anticoagulant that could be taken orally rather than by injection. Warfarin is a more potent derivative of dicoumarol.

water-soluble vitamins include the B vitamins and vitamin C. Thiamin, riboflavin, niacin, biotin, and pantothenic acid are needed as coenzymes in the reactions that produce energy from carbohydrate, fat, and protein. Vitamin B_6 is particularly important for amino acid metabolism. Folate is necessary for DNA synthesis and thus is essential for cell division; adequate intake before and during pregnancy may prevent birth defects called neural tube defects. Vitamin B_{12} is essential for nerve health and for the metabolism of folate and fatty acids. Vitamin C is essential for the health of connective tissue and acts as an antioxidant. The fat-soluble vitamins include vitamins A, D, E, and K. Vitamin A is needed for vision and for the growth and differentiation of cells. Some carotenoids such as β-carotene can be converted into vitamin A. Vitamin D promotes calcium absorption, so it is important for bone health. It can be made in the skin by exposure to sunlight, so if sun exposure is sufficient, it is not needed in the diet. Vitamin E is a fat-soluble antioxidant that protects cell membranes from oxidative damage. Vitamin K is needed for blood clotting.

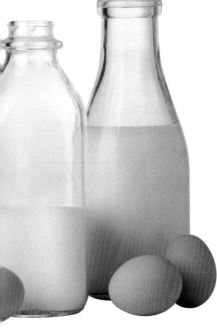

8

Minerals

Minerals—aren't those rocks? Many of the same minerals found in rocks are also found in the human body. The calcium in a limestone cliff, the salt in ocean water, and the iron in your skillet are the same as the calcium in your bones, the salt in your tears, and the iron in your blood. To stay healthy, you need to consume these substances in your diet. Minerals are inorganic elements needed in the diet to provide structure and regulation in the body. Some minerals are an integral part of bone structure; some have very specific roles in transporting oxygen and regulating blood glucose levels. Many minerals serve as **cofactors**, which are **ions** or other molecules required for enzyme activity.

The **major minerals** include sodium, potassium, chloride, calcium, phosphorus, magnesium, and sulfur; they are called major because we need a lot of them—more than 100 mg is needed in the daily diet or they are present in the body in amounts greater than 0.01% of body weight. The **trace elements** are minerals required by the body in an amount of 100 mg or less per day or are present in the body in an amount of 0.01% or less of body weight. They include iron, zinc, copper, manganese, selenium, iodine, chromium, fluoride, and molybdenum. There are also other trace elements found in the body but it has not been determined whether or not they are dietary essentials.

Minerals are found in both plant and animal foods. The mineral content of some foods is predictable because the minerals are regulated components of the plant or animal. For instance, iron is a component of muscle tissue; therefore, it is found in consistent amounts in meat. In other foods, minerals are present as contaminants, so the amounts present vary depending on conditions where the food is produced. For instance, the selenium content of plants depends on the selenium concentration in the soil and water where the plant is grown. Food processing and refining also affect the mineral content of foods. Iron, selenium, zinc, and copper are lost when wheat is refined to make white flour; iron is added when white flour is enriched.

HOW MUCH DO YOU NEED?

The amount of each mineral you need to consume to prevent deficiency and promote health depends on your age, gender, and life stage. Recommendations for mineral intake have been made by the DRIs (Table 8.1). These recommendations must take into account the **bioavailability** of the mineral. Bioavailability is a measure of how much of the mineral is available to the body once the food is eaten. It depends on conditions in your body and constituents of your diet; sometimes these increase the amount available and sometimes they decrease it. For example, more iron is absorbed from the diet when the iron stores in your body are low; calcium is better absorbed in pregnant women when needs are increased. Components of the diet that can reduce mineral absorption include fiber, **phytates, oxalates,** and **tannins.** Fiber is found in grains, fruits, and vegetables; phytates are found in whole grains; oxalates are found in greens and chocolate; and tannins are found in tea and some grains. Foods high in these can reduce mineral absorption. For example, much of the iron in spinach is unavailable because it is bound to oxalates. There are also substances in the diet that promote mineral absorption. For example, including vitamin C in an iron-containing meal can

Table 8.1 Recommended Vitamin Intakes

MINERAL	RECOMMENDED INTAKE FOR ADULTS
Sodium	1500 mg
Potassium	4700 mg
Chloride	2300 mg
Calcium	1000–1200 mg
Phosphorus	700 mg
Magnesium	310–420 mg
Sulfur	None specified
Iron	8–18 mg
Zinc	8–11 mg
Copper	900 µg
Manganese	1.8–2.3 mg
Selenium	55 µg
Iodine	150 µg
Chromium	25–35 µg
Fluoride	3–4 mg
Molybdenum	45 µg

enhance the absorption of iron sixfold. Minerals also interact with each other. For example, a high intake of zinc can reduce copper absorption. All of these interactions tend to balance out in a varied diet and usually do not affect mineral status. However, large doses of mineral supplements may upset the balance, allowing a deficiency or toxicity to occur.

THE ELECTROLYTES: SODIUM, POTASSIUM, AND CHLORIDE

Electrolytes are elements that conduct electricity when dissolved in water. Chemically, many minerals are electrolytes, but in nutrition the term *electrolyte* is used to refer to sodium, potassium, and chloride, the principal electrolytes in body fluids.

Sodium, potassium, and chloride help regulate the amount of fluid in the body and the balance of fluids between different areas or compartments of the body. For example, when the concentration of sodium in the blood increases, water moves into the blood by osmosis, causing an increase in blood volume and blood pressure. The electrolytes are also important for nerve conduction and muscle contraction. Their role in nerve conduction has to do with the distribution of sodium and potassium. Sodium is the most abundant positively charged electrolyte outside cells and potassium is the principal positively charged ion inside cells. At the nerve cell membrane, the number of positively charged ions just outside the membrane is greater than it is inside the membrane. This difference in the electrical charge inside and outside the membrane is called the membrane potential. When a nerve is stimulated, it causes sodium to rush into the cell. This causes a change in the membrane potential that travels along the nerve and is known as a nerve impulse. A similar mechanism causes stimulation of the muscle cell membrane and leads to muscle contraction.

Electrolytes in Our Diets

The modern diet is typically low in potassium and high in sodium. A typical American diet contains about 9 grams of salt; salt is 40% sodium and 60% chloride, so this is equivalent to 3.6 grams of sodium and 5.4 grams of chloride. These amounts are more than double the recommendations of 1.5 and 2.3 grams, respectively. Most of this comes from processed foods. In contrast, we eat less than the recommended amount of potassium (Table 8.1). Most of the potassium in our diet comes from unprocessed foods such as fruits, vegetables, whole grains, and fresh meats.

Electrolyte deficiencies are rare in healthy individuals but may occur as a result of vomiting, diarrhea, increased urinary losses, and excessive sweating. Symptoms include poor appetite, nausea, muscle cramps, confusion, apathy, constipation, and irregular heartbeat. Electrolyte toxicity is also rare; it does occur when supplements are consumed in excess or when kidney function is compromised.

Balancing Electrolytes in and out

The intake of sodium varies greatly among different populations. For example, in northern China, sodium chloride intake is greater than 13.9 grams per day, while in the Kalahari Desert, it is less than 1.7 grams per day. Nonetheless, blood levels of sodium are not significantly different among these groups. This is because levels of electrolytes are closely regulated.

Sodium and chloride levels in the body are regulated by the intake of both water and salt. When salt intake is high, thirst is stimulated to increase water intake. When salt intake is very low, a salt appetite causes the individual to seek out salt. These mechanisms help ensure that appropriate proportions of salt and water are consumed. The kidneys, however, are the primary regulator of sodium, chloride, and potassium balance in the body. Excretion of sodium in the urine is decreased when intake is low and increased when intake is high. Because water follows sodium by osmosis, the ability of the kidneys to conserve sodium provides a mechanism to conserve body water.

Changes in the amount of sodium in the blood affect blood pressure, and changes in blood pressure trigger the production and release of proteins and hormones that alter the amount of sodium, and hence water, retained by the kidneys. A decrease in blood pressure leads to the release of the hormone aldosterone, which acts on the kidneys to increase sodium and chloride reabsorption. Water follows the reabsorbed sodium, resulting in an increase in blood volume and, consequently, blood pressure.

As with sodium and chloride, the kidneys regulate potassium excretion to maintain a relatively constant amount of potassium in the body. If blood levels begin to rise, mechanisms are activated to stimulate the cellular uptake of potassium. This short-term regulation prevents the amount of potassium in the extracellular fluid from getting lethally high. The long-term regulation of potassium balance depends on aldosterone release, which causes the kidney to excrete potassium and retain sodium.

Electrolytes and Blood Pressure

Blood pressure is the pressure that the blood exerts against blood vessels. Normal blood pressure is less than 120/80 mm of mercury. Blood pressure increases when blood volume is too high or the blood vessels become narrow and inelastic. High blood pressure, known as **hypertension**, is defined as a blood pressure that is consistently 140/90 mm of mercury or greater. Hypertension increases the risk of atherosclerosis, heart attack, stroke, and kidney disease.

The cause of most cases of hypertension is not known, but a family history of hypertension, excess body weight, lack of exercise, and certain dietary patterns increase risk. Diets high in salt are associated with a higher incidence of hypertension, whereas diets high in fiber, potassium, calcium, and magnesium are associated with a lower incidence of hypertension. The recommendation to keep sodium intake below 1.5 g per day is based on the fact that a high intake of sodium may cause an increase in blood pressure. Because there are many dietary factors involved in blood pressure regulation, the **DASH diet** (Dietary Approaches to Stop Hypertension), is recommended to keep blood pressure in the normal range. This dietary pattern is high in fruits, vegetables, low-fat dairy products, whole grains, and lean meats, making it high in potassium, calcium, magnesium, and fiber, and moderate in salt and fat.

CALCIUM

Drink your milk. Children hear it from their mothers and adults hear it from their doctors. They hear it because milk is an excellent source of calcium. Calcium is needed for the development and maintenance of strong healthy bones. If calcium intake is low in childhood, the bones may not achieve their maximum strength. If intake is low in adulthood, bone strength may be lost more quickly than is normal. In either case, the result may be an increase in bone fractures later in life.

Calcium is the most abundant mineral in the body. It is important for the maintenance of bones and teeth where it is part of a solid crystalline material called hydroxyapatite. It also plays extremely important roles in cell communication and the regulation of body processes. It is needed to release neurotransmitters so that a nerve signal can pass from a nerve to the target cell. Inside the muscle cells, the presence of calcium allows the two muscle proteins, actin and myosin, to interact to cause muscle contraction. Calcium also plays a role in blood pressure regulation and blood clotting.

Getting Calcium Into Your Body

Most of the calcium in the American diet comes from dairy products such as milk, cheese, and yogurt. Other good sources include tofu, legumes, leafy green vegetables, and fish that are consumed with the bones, such as sardines. Foods fortified with calcium such as breakfast cereals and juices also make an important contribution to the calcium content of the American diet.

The amount of calcium absorbed from the diet depends on vitamin D status, life stage, and other dietary components. Although some calcium can be absorbed in the absence of vitamin D, vitamin D-dependent absorption accounts for most of the calcium absorbed when intakes are low to moderate. Calcium absorption is increased when calcium need is high, such as during infancy and pregnancy. Calcium absorption is increased by the presence of the sugar lactose but is reduced by the presence of fiber, phytates from whole grains, and oxalates from foods such as spinach, sweet potatoes, and rhubarb. Chocolate also contains oxalates, but chocolate milk is still a good source of calcium.

Regulating Calcium Levels

Maintaining calcium homeostasis is critical to nerve transmission and muscle contraction, and hence survival. Even small changes in blood calcium levels trigger regulatory mechanisms. The hormones parathyroid hormone (PTH), which raises blood calcium, and **calcitonin**, which lowers blood calcium, are key to calcium regulation.

When blood calcium levels drop, PTH is released from the parathyroid gland and acts in three different ways to raise blood calcium levels. At the bone, it stimulates bone breakdown to release calcium; at the kidney, it reduces calcium excretion so more is retained in the blood; and also at the kidney, it signals the activation of vitamin D. Active vitamin D then enhances the absorption of

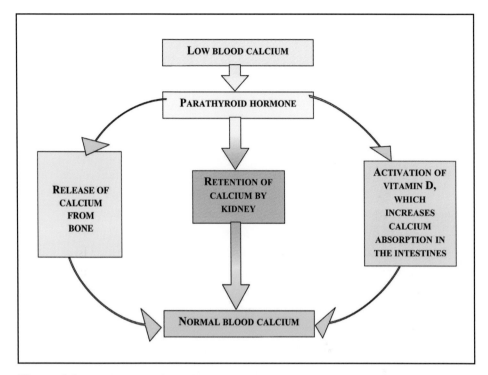

Figure 8.1 Low blood calcium stimulates the release of parathyroid hormone, which acts to return blood calcium to normal.

dietary calcium from the intestine (Figure 8.1). When blood calcium levels rise, the release of PTH is stopped and the hormone calcitonin is released from the thyroid gland. Calcitonin acts on the bone to inhibit the release of calcium, resulting in a decrease in blood calcium levels.

Calcium and Health: Osteoporosis

The ability to maintain blood calcium levels by removing calcium from bone prevents life-threatening drops in blood calcium and is therefore beneficial over the short term. However, if continued over the long term, it results in weakened bones that are susceptible to fractures. This condition is known as **osteoporosis**. Osteoporosis is an important public health concern in the United States, where about

44 million people aged 50 or over have osteoporosis or are at risk due to low bone mass. Osteoporosis is estimated to cause 1.5 million fractures annually.

The risk of developing osteoporosis depends on how dense the bones are and the balance between bone formation and bone breakdown. Bone is active living tissue that is constantly being broken down and reformed. In growing children, bone formation occurs more rapidly than breakdown. Bone deposition continues to outpace bone breakdown into young adulthood when **peak bone mass** is achieved. After about age 35 to 40, bone breakdown exceeds formation, so bone is slowly lost and bone density declines. If a high peak bone mass has been achieved, the loss of bone that occurs later in life will not leave bones so depleted that fractures occur.

The risk of osteoporosis depends on age, gender, genetics, diet, and lifestyle. Risk increases with age. Osteoporosis is more common in women than men and more common in Caucasians than in African Americans. The most significant dietary factor contributing to osteoporosis is low calcium intake during the years of bone formation. Diets high in phytates, oxalates, and tannins or low in vitamin D reduce calcium absorption and may contribute to

---

FACT BOX 8.1

How Common Is Osteoporosis?

In the United States, it is estimated that approximately 8 million women aged 50 and over have osteoporosis and another 22 million have low bone mass, which increases the risk of osteoporosis. The incidence of this disease is lower in men but it is still estimated that more than 2 million men 50 years of age and older have osteoporosis and almost 12 million have low bone mass. Therefore, in the United States, osteoporosis and low bone mass threaten almost 44 million American adults, or 55% of people 50 and older. If current trends continue, more than 52 million men and women in this age group will be affected by the year 2010 and this figure will to climb to over 61 million by 2020.

From: "America's Bone Health: The State of Osteoporosis and Low Bone Mass." National Osteoporosis Association. Available online at *http://www.nof.org/advocacy/prevalence/index.htm*.

a low peak bone mass. Adequate dietary protein is necessary for bone health, and higher intakes of zinc, magnesium, potassium, fiber, and vitamin C are associated with greater bone mass.[22] Lifestyle factors that affect the risk of osteoporosis include cigarette smoking and excessive alcohol consumption, which decrease peak bone mass, and weight-bearing exercise, which increases peak bone mass. The risk of osteoporosis can be minimized by a lifelong diet rich in fruits and vegetables, adequate in calcium and vitamin D, and not excessive in phosphorus, protein, or sodium. Individuals who do not meet their calcium needs with diet alone can benefit from calcium supplementation. Once osteoporosis has developed, it is difficult to restore lost bone.

Excessive calcium consumption occurs primarily from the use of supplements. Too much calcium may cause kidney stones in susceptible individuals, and may interfere with the absorption of other minerals.

PHOSPHORUS

Phosphorus is an important structural component of bones where, along with calcium, it forms mineral crystals called hydroxapatite. Phosphorus also has other structural and regulatory roles. It is a component of phospholipids, which make up the basic structure of cell membranes. It is a major constituent of DNA and RNA and is important in energy transfers because the high-energy bonds of ATP are formed between phosphate groups. Phosphorus, as phosphate, also acts as a buffer to regulate the level of acidity in cells.

Phosphorus is found in a wide range of foods. These include dairy products, meat, fish, cereals, eggs, and nuts. Food additives used in baked goods, cheeses, processed meats, and soft drinks also provide phosphorus. Unlike calcium, vitamin D does not need to be available to absorb adequate amounts of phosphorus.

To support bone mineralization, blood levels of phosphorus must be balanced with calcium levels. This balance is maintained through the actions of vitamin D and parathyroid hormone (PTH). When blood levels of phosphorus are low, the active form of vitamin D is synthesized, increasing phosphorus and calcium absorption from the intestine and releasing it from bone. A rise in serum phosphorus indirectly stimulates PTH release, causing phosphorus excretion and calcium retention by the kidney. When PTH is not secreted, phosphorus is retained and calcium is excreted in the urine.

Phosphorus deficiency can affect bone health but is rare because this mineral is so widely distributed in foods. The increased use of phosphorus-containing food additives has created concern about excessive phosphorus intake, which can cause bone breakdown. These higher levels of phosphorus are not believed to affect bone health as long as calcium is adequate.

MAGNESIUM

Magnesium is a component of the green plant pigment chlorophyll, so leafy green vegetables are a good dietary source. Whole grains, nuts, and seeds are also good sources. About half of the magnesium in the diet is absorbed. Absorption is enhanced by the active form of vitamin D and decreased by the presence of phytates and calcium.

Magnesium has many diverse roles throughout the body. It is less plentiful in bone than calcium and phosphorus but is still essential for the maintenance of bone structure. It is involved in regulating calcium homeostasis and is needed for the action of vitamin D and several hormones. It is also a cofactor for enzymes involved in energy production from carbohydrate, lipid, and protein. It is essential for maintenance of electrical potentials across cell membranes and proper functioning of the nerves and muscles, including those in the heart. It is important for the synthesis of protein, DNA, and RNA and is needed to stabilize ATP structure. Magnesium may also be involved in blood pressure regulation.

The kidneys regulate blood levels of magnesium so homeostasis can be maintained over a wide range of dietary intakes. Magnesium deficiency is rare but may occur in individuals with alcoholism, malnutrition, and kidney or intestinal disease; symptoms include nausea, muscle weakness and cramping, irritability, mental derangement, and changes in blood pressure and heartbeat. Toxic effects have not been observed from ingestion of magnesium in foods, but toxicity may occur from concentrated sources such as magnesium-containing drugs and supplements. Magnesium toxicity is characterized by nausea, vomiting, low blood pressure, and other cardiovascular changes.

SULFUR

Sulfur is a component of many essential substances in the body. Thiamin and biotin contain sulfur in their structure. It is also part of glutathione, which is important in detoxifying drugs and protecting cells from oxidative damage. Methionine and cysteine are sulfur-containing amino acids. Sulfur-containing ions are a part of an important buffer system that regulates acid-base balance. Sulfur in the diet comes from the sulfur-containing amino acids in proteins, some sulfur-containing vitamins, and inorganic sulfur compounds used as food preservatives. There is no recommended intake for sulfur, and no deficiencies are known when protein needs are met.

IRON

Are you tired? Irritable? Having trouble concentrating? You may just need a good night's sleep, or you may be suffering from iron deficiency, the most common nutritional deficiency in this country and around the world.

What Does Iron Do?

Iron is needed for the delivery of oxygen to cells. Most of the iron in the body is part of hemoglobin, the protein that gives red blood cells their red color. Hemoglobin transports oxygen to body cells and carries carbon dioxide away from cells for elimination by the lungs. Iron is also a component of the muscle protein myoglobin, which stores oxygen for use in the muscle. Iron is part of an enzyme in the citric acid cycle and several proteins involved in the electron transport chain. It is needed for the activity of catalase, an enzyme that protects cells from oxidative damage. Iron-containing proteins are also involved in drug metabolism and the immune system.

Iron in Our Diet

Iron comes from both animal and plant sources. Much of the iron in animal products is part of a chemical complex called heme.

Heme iron is easily absorbed and is plentiful in meat, poultry, and fish. Plant sources of iron contain only **nonheme iron**, which is not as well absorbed. Sources include leafy green vegetables, legumes, and grains. Nonheme iron also leaches into food from iron cooking utensils such as iron skillets. Heme iron absorption is not affected by other components of the diet but the proportion of nonheme iron that is absorbed varies depending on the foods consumed with the iron. It is better absorbed in the presence of acids and heme iron; vitamin C enhances absorption because it is an acid and because it forms a complex with iron that improves its absorption. Fiber, phytates, tannins, and oxalates reduce absorption. The presence of other minerals may also decrease iron absorption.

Regulating Iron Levels

Iron is not easily eliminated from the body. Even when red blood cells die, the iron in their hemoglobin is not lost, but recycled to make new red blood cells. Therefore, the amount of iron in the body is controlled by regulating how much is transported from the GI tract into the body. The amount of iron transported from the mucosal cells of the intestine to the rest of the body depends on need. When body iron is in short supply, the iron transport protein, **transferrin**, is able to pick up more iron from the intestines and deliver it to body cells. When iron is plentiful in the body, more of the iron storage protein **ferritin** is made. This increases the amount of iron bound to ferritin in the intestinal mucosal cells and reduces the amount of iron transported to other body cells. Iron that remains bound to ferritin in the mucosal cells is excreted in the feces when these cells die. Some of the iron that is transported from the intestine is stored in the liver bound to ferritin. When ferritin concentrations in the liver become high, some is converted to an insoluble iron storage protein called hemosiderin.

Iron and Anemia

In the United States, iron deficiency affects 7.8 million adolescent girls and women of childbearing age and 700,000 children aged one to two years. When iron is deficient, hemoglobin cannot be made

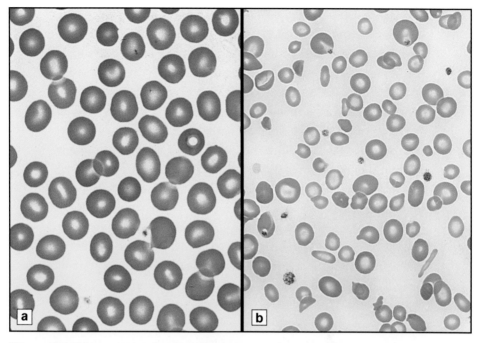

Figure 8.2 When someone has iron deficiency anemia, red blood cells are smaller and paler than normal because they do not contain as much hemoglobin. Normal human red blood cells are shown on the left (a) and anemic red blood cells are shown on the right (b).

and the red blood cells that are formed are small and pale and unable to deliver adequate oxygen to the tissues (Figure 8.2). This condition is known as iron deficiency anemia. Symptoms of iron deficiency anemia include fatigue, weakness, headache, decreased work capacity, an inability to maintain body temperature in a cold environment, changes in behavior, decreased resistance to infection, impaired development in infants, and an increased risk of lead poisoning in young children.

Groups at risk of iron deficiency include women of reproductive age, pregnant women, infants, adolescents, and athletes. Women of reproductive age are at risk for iron deficiency anemia because of iron loss due to menstruation. Pregnant women are at risk because iron needs increase to expand maternal blood volume and allow the growth of other maternal tissues and the fetus. Infants and adolescents are at risk because their rapid growth increases iron needs. Athletes are susceptible to iron deficiency because prolonged training increases losses and some athletes do not consume enough in their diets.

Too Much Iron Can Be Deadly

Even though iron is essential for health, it can also be deadly. Ingestion of a single large dose damages the intestinal lining, alters body acidity, and can cause shock and liver failure. Iron supplement overdose is the most common form of poisoning in children less than six years of age. Too much body iron, or iron overload, can occur in individuals who require frequent transfusions but the most common cause is **hemochromatosis**. This is a genetic condition that allows increased iron absorption. The accumulation of excess iron that occurs in hemochromatosis causes heart and liver damage, diabetes, and certain types of cancer. Iron deposits also darken the skin.

FACT BOX 8.2

Hemochromatosis

Hemochromatosis is the most common inherited disease in Caucasian populations in North America, Australia, and Europe. In the United States it affects 1.5 million people, about 1 in 300 individuals. Treatment of this disorder will prevent the complications of iron overload and is simple— regular blood withdrawal. Unfortunately, many people do not know they have hemochromatosis until organ damage has already occurred. The availability of red meat, the enrichment of grain products with iron, and the abundance of iron-fortified foods in our food supply just about guarantees that those with this disease who are not being treated will eventually accumulate damaging amounts of iron. To be effective, treatment must begin before organs are damaged, so early identification of people with this disease is essential in preventing complications.[a] The gene for hemochromatosis has been identified and genetic testing is available.[b]

a Edwards, C.Q., Griffin, L.M., Ajioka, R.S., and Kushner, J.P. "Screening for Hemochromatosis: Phenotype Versus Genotype." *Seminars in Hematology* 35: 72–76, 1998.

b Hollan, S. "Iron Overload in Light of the Identification of a Haemochromatosis Gene." *Haematologia* 28: 109–116, 1997.

ZINC

In an alphabetical list zinc may come last but it is the second most common trace metal in the body, after iron. Zinc is involved in the functioning of nearly 100 different enzymes. It is vital in protecting cells from **free radical** damage. It is needed for the activity of enzymes that function in the synthesis of DNA and RNA, in carbohydrate metabolism, in acid-base balance, and in a reaction that is necessary for folate absorption. It plays a role in the storage and release of insulin, the mobilization of vitamin A from the liver, and the stabilization of cell membranes. Zinc is important in **gene expression** and therefore is needed for the growth and repair of tissues, the activity of the immune system, and the development of sex organs and bone. Zinc-containing proteins are needed for the activity of vitamin A, vitamin D, and a number of hormones including thyroid hormones, estrogen, and testosterone. Without zinc, these nutrients and hormones cannot bind to DNA to increase or decrease gene expression and, hence, the synthesis of certain proteins.

Zinc is found in red meat, liver, eggs, dairy products, vegetables, and some seafood. Whole grains are a good source but refined grains are not, because zinc is lost in milling and not added back in enrichment. Grain products leavened with yeast provide more zinc than unleavened products because the yeast leavening of breads reduces the phytate content.[23]

Severe zinc deficiency is rare in North America but is a problem in developing countries. It has been reported in populations that consume diets based on cereal proteins from which zinc is poorly absorbed. Symptoms include poor growth and development, skin rashes, and decreased immune function. Moderate zinc deficiency is more of a concern in the United States. A moderate zinc deficiency causes a decrease in the number and function of immune cells in the blood and therefore can lead to an increased incidence of infections.

High intakes of zinc can impair immune function, increase the risk of heart disease, and interfere with copper absorption. Zinc is often marketed as a supplement to improve immune function, enhance fertility and sexual performance, and cure the common cold. Supplements have been shown to reduce the incidence of diarrhea and infections in deficient individuals, but there is no evidence that extra is beneficial. Over-supplementation may result in toxicity.

COPPER

It is logical that too little iron in your diet can cause iron deficiency anemia, but did you know that too little copper can also cause iron deficiency anemia? This can occur because copper is a component of the protein **ceruloplasmin**, which converts iron into a form that can bind to transferrin for transport. If copper is deficient, iron cannot be transported and an iron deficiency occurs. Copper is also needed for the function of a number of proteins and enzymes that are involved in iron and lipid metabolism, connective tissue synthesis, maintenance of heart muscle, and function of the immune and central nervous systems.[24] It is needed for the synthesis of the neurotransmitters norepinephrine and dopamine, the pigment melanin, and several blood clotting factors. Copper is also an essential component of a form of the antioxidant enzyme superoxide dismutase.

Dietary sources of copper include organ meats, seafood, nuts and seeds, whole grains, and chocolate. Only about 30% to 40% of the copper in a typical diet is absorbed. Copper absorption is enhanced by amino acids and reduced by high intakes of zinc, iron, manganese, molybdenum, and vitamin C.

Copper deficiency is relatively rare and not a problem in North America where the amount of copper in the diet is slightly above the RDA. It has been documented in premature infants and in patients fed intravenous solutions lacking copper. In addition to iron deficiency anemia, copper deficiency may cause impaired growth, degeneration of the heart muscle, degeneration of the nervous system, and changes in hair color and structure. Because of copper's role in the development and maintenance of the immune system, a diet low in copper decreases the immune response and increases the incidence of infection. Copper toxicity from dietary sources is rare.

MANGANESE

Only about 10 to 20 milligrams of manganese is present in the body, but it is a key component of some enzymes and an activator of others. Manganese-requiring enzymes are involved in amino acid, carbohydrate, and cholesterol metabolism; cartilage formation; urea synthesis; and antioxidant protection. Like copper and zinc, manganese protects against oxidative damage by functioning in a form of superoxide dismutase.

The best dietary sources of manganese are whole grains, legumes, nuts, and tea. Manganese absorption increases when intake is low and decreases when intake is high. It is eliminated from the body by excretion into the intestinal tract in bile.

A naturally occurring manganese deficiency has never been reported in humans. Toxicity causes nerve damage and has been reported due to industrial exposure, rather than dietary intake.

SELENIUM

In the early 1930s, selenium was identified as the toxic agent that caused lameness and death in livestock that ate certain plants. About 25 years later, this trace element was recognized as an essential nutrient. Selenium is important in the body's antioxidant defenses. It is an essential part of the enzyme glutathione peroxidase, which helps neutralize compounds called peroxides so they no longer form free radicals and cause oxidative damage. By reducing free radical formation, selenium can spare some of the need for the antioxidant vitamin E. Selenium is also needed for the synthesis of the thyroid hormones, which regulate metabolic rate.

Dietary sources of selenium include seafood, kidney, liver, and eggs. Grains can be a good source of selenium, depending on the selenium content of the soil where they are grown. Because of this, soil selenium content can have a significant impact on the selenium intake of populations consuming primarily locally grown food.

Selenium deficiency causes muscle discomfort and weakness. It is uncommon but has been identified in individuals receiving intravenous solutions lacking selenium and in regions of China where the soil is deficient in selenium and the people consume only locally grown food. In China, selenium deficiency is associated with a form of heart disease called Keshan disease. Although selenium supplements relieve most of the symptoms of Keshan disease and reduce its incidence, selenium deficiency is not the only cause of this disease.[25] Low intakes of selenium have also been associated with an increased incidence of certain types of cancer.

Dietary toxicity occurs in regions of China with very high soil selenium levels and has been reported in the United States because of an error in the manufacture of a supplement. Symptoms include hair loss, fingernail loss, and gastrointestinal upset.

IODINE

Did you ever wonder what iodized salt is? Iodized salt is salt that has been fortified with iodine. Fortification of salt with iodine began in the 1920s because iodine deficiency was a serious public health problem in the central part of the United States and Canada. The most obvious outward sign of iodine deficiency is an enlarged thyroid gland called a goiter (Figure 8.3). A goiter forms because iodine is needed for the production of thyroid hormones, which regulate basal metabolic rate, growth, and development, and promote protein synthesis. When iodine is deficient, levels of thyroid hormones drop. When they drop, the thyroid gland tries to fix the problem by making more thyroid hormones. Because iodine is unavailable, the thyroid hormones cannot be made, yet the thyroid gland continues to be stimulated. The continuous stimulation causes the thyroid gland to enlarge.

Natural dietary sources of iodine include seafood and plants grown close to the sea where the iodine content of the soil is high. Iodine-containing food contaminants and food additives also contribute to the iodine content of the American diet. However, most of the iodine in the American diet comes from iodized salt.

Iodine deficiency can occur due to a low iodine intake or the consumption of a diet high in goitrogens, substances in turnips, rutabaga, cabbage, and cassava that interfere with the utilization of iodine or with thyroid function. When iodine is deficient, adequate amounts of the thyroid hormones cannot be made causing metabolic rate to slow. This results in fatigue and weight gain. Goiter is only one of the iodine deficiency disorders. The deficiency also increases the risk of spontaneous abortion in pregnant women and can cause a birth defect know as **cretinism** in the offspring.

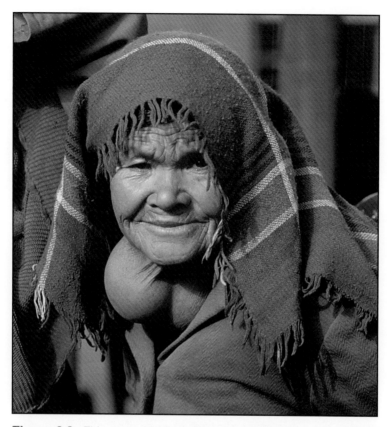

Figure 8.3 This women has a goiter—an enlargement of the thyroid gland. A goiter is one of the symptoms of iodine deficiency.

Cretinism is characterized by mental retardation, deafness, and growth failure. Because of the fortification of table salt with iodine, cretinism and goiter are now rare in North America but iodine deficiency remains a world health problem. Salt iodinization programs are under way in most countries where an iodine deficiency is a public health issue.[26] For groups who do not use iodized salt, other forms of iodine supplementation, such as injections or oral doses of iodized oil, may be effective for control of iodine deficiency.[27] High intakes of iodine can cause an enlargement of the thyroid gland that resembles goiter, so levels of fortification and supplementation should be monitored.

CHROMIUM

Wouldn't it be great if you could take a pill that would decrease your body fat and increase the amount of muscle you have? The dietary supplement chromium picolinate claims to do just that. Unfortunately, studies examining chromium picolinate have found it to have no beneficial effects on muscle strength, body composition, or weight loss.[28] Chromium is, however, important for the uptake of glucose by cells and other actions of the hormone insulin. Chromium acts by stabilizing insulin and amplifying its effects. When chromium is deficient, it takes more insulin to keep blood glucose in the normal range.

Dietary sources include liver, nuts, and whole grains. Chromium intake can be increased by cooking in stainless steel cookware because chromium leaches from the steel into the food.

Deficiencies have been reported in patients fed intravenous solutions devoid of chromium and in malnourished children. Deficiency symptoms include impaired glucose tolerance with diabetes-like symptoms, such as elevated blood glucose levels and increased insulin levels.

FLUORIDE

Do you use a fluoride toothpaste? Fluoride is added to toothpaste because brushing it on your teeth helps prevent cavities. Fluoride consumed in the diet also helps prevent tooth decay. This is because it is incorporated into the enamel crystals of teeth, making them more resistant to the acid that causes decay. Fluoride is also important for bone health. Fluoride has its greatest effect on dental caries prevention early in life, during maximum tooth development (up to the age of 13), but it has also been shown to have beneficial effects in adults.[29] Because it is so important for dental health, it has been added to some municipal water supplies since the 1940s. Today, over half of the population of the United States lives in communities with fluoridated drinking water.

Most of the fluoride in our diet comes from fluoridated water and from fluoride added to toothpaste. Natural sources include tea and marine fish. Excess intakes of fluoride can cause mottled teeth in children and extremely high doses can be deadly. Because of this, toothpaste now carries a warning that it should not be swallowed.

MOLYBDENUM

Molybdenum is needed to activate enzymes involved in the metabolism of sulfur-containing amino acids, nitrogen-containing compounds present in DNA and RNA, uric acid production, and the detoxification of other compounds. It is consumed in milk, milk products, organ meats, breads, cereals, and legumes. Deficiency is rare but has been reported in individuals fed intravenous solutions for long periods of time.

CONNECTIONS

Minerals are elements needed by the body to provide structure and regulation. The bioavailability of minerals depends on the needs of the body as well as interactions with other constituents in the diet. The electrolytes sodium, potassium, and chloride are needed for fluid balance and nerve conduction. A high-sodium diet may contribute to hypertension. Calcium is needed for nerve transmission and muscle contraction and, along with phosphorus, forms the hard mineral deposits in bones and teeth. Magnesium is also important for bone health and is a cofactor for enzymes involved in energy production from carbohydrate, lipid, and protein. Iron is part of hemoglobin, which transports oxygen in the blood, and it is a component of a number of proteins needed for energy production. Iron deficiency anemia is common in the United States and around the world. Zinc is needed for tissue growth and repair, immune function, and antioxidant protection. Copper is needed for iron transport, connective tissue health, and antioxidant protection. Manganese is needed for the activity of a number of enzymes, including one involved in antioxidant defenses. Selenium is also needed for the activity of an antioxidant enzyme system. Iodine is a component of the thyroid hormones that regulate metabolic rate, growth, and development. Chromium is needed for the action of insulin. Fluoride is important for strong tooth enamel. Molybdenum is a coenzyme important in amino acid metabolism.

9

Choosing a Healthy Diet

Knowing what nutrients are and how much of each is recommended for optimal health is important. However, this information is not always helpful in choosing a healthy diet. Because of the wide variety of foods available to us today, there are many ways in which you can choose healthy diet. Virtually any food can be part of a healthy diet as long as it is balanced with other food choices throughout the day or week to meet but not exceed needs.

WHAT IS A HEALTHY DIET?

A healthy diet is one that provides the right number of calories to keep your weight in the desirable range; the proper balance of carbohydrate, protein, and fat choices; plenty of water; and sufficient but not excessive amounts of essential vitamins and minerals. Generally, recommendations from the Food Guide Pyramid and the Dietary Guidelines suggest a diet that is rich in whole grains, fruits, and vegetables; high in fiber; moderate in fat and sodium; and low in saturated fat, cholesterol, *trans* fat, and added sugars. Choosing this diet does not mean giving up your favorite foods. But it does require considering variety and balance.

Choosing a variety of foods is important because even within food groups different foods provide different nutrients. For example, strawberries are a fruit that provide vitamin C but little vitamin A, whereas apricots provide a source of vitamin A, but less vitamin C. If you choose only strawberries, you will get plenty of vitamin C but may be lacking in vitamin A. Balancing your diet means choosing foods that complement each other. This requires considering the nutrient density of foods you choose. Foods low in nutrient density such as baked goods, snack foods, and sodas should be balanced with nutrient-dense choices such as salads, fresh fruit, and large vegetable servings. For one meal you may choose a burger, french fries, and a milkshake; you can balance this with a salad, brown rice, and chicken at the next meal.

No single dietary component can make or break a diet. Rather, it is the overall pattern of dietary intake combined with lifestyle factors that determines the relationship between your diet and your health. For example, the diet in Italy and other Mediterranean countries is higher in fat than the U.S. diet, yet the people's incidence of heart disease is lower than ours. This is thought to be related to the fact that much of the fat in this Mediterranean diet is monounsaturated fat from olive oil and, in addition, their diet is higher in fruits and vegetables and their lifestyle is less stressful than ours.

MAINTAINING A HEALTHY WEIGHT

A healthy body weight is associated with health and longevity. Maintaining a healthy weight means matching the calories you consume in your diet with the energy you expend to stay alive and active. Unfortunately, many Americans consume more calories than they burn and are consequently overweight or obese.

How Many Calories Do You Need?

The number of calories you need depends on how many calories your body uses. Your body needs energy to stay alive, to keep your heart beating, your kidneys working, and your body warm. It needs energy to digest the food you eat and process the nutrients it contains. It also needs energy to fuel activity. Your calorie needs can be estimated by calculating your estimated energy requirement (EER) using an equation that takes into account your age, gender, height, weight, and activity level. To estimate your calorie needs, start

---

FACT BOX 9.1

Has Okinawa Found the Fountain of Youth?

In Okinawa, almost 29% of the population lives to be 100. That's nearly 4 times the average number in the West. Life expectancy in Okinawa, a series of islands between mainland Japan and Taiwan, is 81.2 years. In the United States, life expectancy is 76.8 years. In addition to the longest life expectancy in the world, Okinawa has the lowest rates of heart disease, cancer, and stroke, giving the nation the world's greatest health expectancy. How do the Okinawans do it? Have they found the elusive fountain of youth?

A major contributor to their long, healthy lives may be Hara Hachi Bu. Hara Hachi Bu is the practice of eating only until you are 80% full. Research in animals has shown that restricting calorie intake can extend life span. Perhaps this is also the case with Okinawans. Their reduced intake allows elder Okinawans to remain lean; they typically have a body mass index (BMI) between 18 and 22, whereas the typical BMI for adults over 60 years of age in the United States is between 26 and 27.

Other factors that are thought to contribute to this long, healthy life are an active lifestyle, a low-stress environment, and a moderate diet that is high in soy, vegetables, and fish, and low in salt and alcohol. Okinawa has a warm climate, so fresh vegetables are available year-round. Their diet is rich in unrefined complex carbohydrates and tofu, which is made from soybeans. Pork is an important part of the diet but the meat is boiled for hours and the fat drained off before it is eaten. A research study called the Okinawan Centenarian Study, which began in 1976, is still ongoing to try to identify the genetic, dietary, and lifestyle factors that contribute to healthy aging in Okinawa.

From: Okinawa Centenarian Study. Available online at *http://okinawaprogram.com/study.html.*

by estimating how active you are. A "sedentary" individual is one who does not participate in any activity beyond that required for daily independent living, such as housework, homework, yard work, gardening, and walking the dog. To be in the "low active" category, an adult weighing 70 kg would need to expend an amount of energy equivalent to walking 2.2 miles at a rate of 3 to 4 miles per hour in addition to the activities of daily living. To be "active," this adult would need to perform daily exercise equivalent to walking 7 miles at a rate of 3 to 4 miles per hour, and to be "very active," he or she would need to perform the equivalent of walking 17 miles at this rate in addition to the activities of daily living. After you have determined your activity level, you can calculate your calorie needs using the equations in Table 9.1.

What Is a Healthy Weight for You?

The current standard for body weight is **body mass index**, or **BMI**. BMI is a ratio of weight to height calculated by the following mathematical equation:

$$BMI = weight\ in\ kg/(height\ in\ m)^2\ or,$$

$$BMI = weight\ in\ pounds/(height\ in\ inches)^2\ x\ 703.$$

For example, someone who is 6 feet (72 inches) tall and weighs 180 pounds has a body mass index of 24.4 kg/m^2 (180/72^2 x 703). For children and young adults, a healthy BMI is defined by where BMI for age falls on the growth charts (Appendix C). For boys, a weight between the 85th and 95th percentiles is considered at risk for overweight and a BMI over the 95th percentile is considered over-weight (Figure 9.1). For individuals over the age of 20, a healthy body weight is defined as a BMI between 18.5 and 24.9 kg/m^2. In general, people with a BMI within this range have the fewest health risks. Underweight is defined as a body mass index of less than 18.5 kg/m^2, overweight is defined as 25 to 29.9 kg/m^2, and obese is 30 kg/m^2 or greater.[30] A BMI of 40 or over is classified as extreme or morbid obesity.

Table 9.1 Calculating Your Calorie Needs

- Determine your weight in kilograms (kg) and your height in meters (m)

   Weight in kg = weight in pounds / 2.2 pounds per kg

   Height in meters = height in inches x 0.0254 inches per m

For example:

   160 pounds = 160 lbs/2.2 lbs/kg = 72.7 kg

   5 feet 9 inches = 69 inches x 0.0254 in/m = 1.75 m

- Estimate your physical activity level and find your PA value in the table below.

LIFE STAGE	PHYSICAL ACTIVITY FACTOR (PA)			
Activity Level	Sedentary	Low Active	Active	Very Active
Boys 3–18 yrs	1	1.13	1.26	1.42
Girls 3–18 yrs	1	1.16	1.31	1.56
Men	1	1.11	1.25	1.48
Women	1	1.12	1.27	1.45

   For example, if you are an active 19-year-old male, your PA value is 1.25.

- Use the appropriate EER prediction equation below to find your EER:

For example:

   If you are an active 19-year-old male,

   EER = 662 – (9.53 x Age in yrs) + PA [(15.91 x Weight in kg) + (539.6 x Height in m)]

   Where age = 19 yr, weight = 72.7 kg, height = 1.75 m, Active PA =1.25

   EER = 662 – (9.53 x 19)+ 1.25 [(15.91 x 72.7) + (539.6 x 1.75)] = 3,107 cal/day

LIFE STAGE	EER PREDICTION EQUATION
Boys 9–18 yrs	EER = 88.5 – (61.9 x Age in yrs) + PA [(26.7 x Weight in kg) + (903 x Height in m)] + 25
Girls 9–18 yrs	EER = 135.3 – (30.8 x Age in yrs) + PA [(10.0 x Weight in kg) + (934 x Height in m)] + 25
Men ≥19 yrs	EER = 662 – (9.53 x Age in yrs) + PA [(15.91 x Weight in kg) + (539.6 x Height in m)]
Women ≥19 yrs	EER = 354 – (6.91 x Age in yrs) + PA [(9.36 x Weight in kg) + (726 x Height in m)]

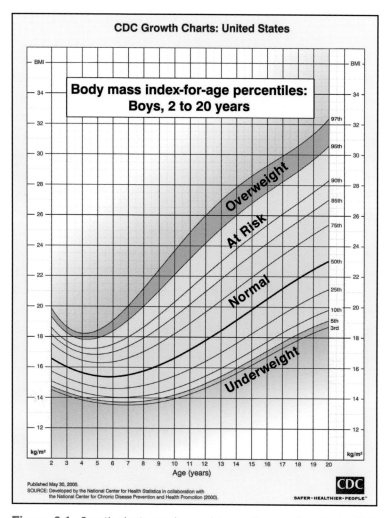

Figure 9.1 Growth charts can be used to monitor growth patterns. This example illustrates BMI-for-age percentiles for males 2 to 20. The colored areas represent BMI values that are associated with underweight, normal weight, at risk of overweight, and overweight. (National Center for Health Statistics, National Center for Chronic Disease Prevention and Health Promotion, 2000.)

An Obesity Epidemic

Today, over 63% of adults in the United States are overweight or obese.[31] The prevalence of obesity is increasing at an alarming rate; it went from 23.3% in 1991 to 30.9% today, an increase of almost

8% in the last decade. Although obesity has increased in both men and women and in every age group and culture in the nation, disparities still exist. More women (33%) are obese than men (28%). The problem is worse among non-Hispanic black women (50%) and Mexican-American women (40%) than in non-Hispanic white women (30%). Weight problems are also increasing among children and adolescents. Ten percent of children between 2 and 5 years of age are overweight and 15% of children and teens 6 to 19 years of age are at risk for being overweight.

Why are we getting fatter? The simple answer is that we are eating more calories than we are burning. When the calories we eat are equal to calories we expend, our weight remains stable. When we eat less than we expend, we lose weight, and when we eat more than we expend, we get fatter. One reason people in the United States today are getting fatter is our ready supply of palatable, affordable food available 24 hours a day in supermarkets, fast-food restaurants, and all-night convenience marts. Another reason is that we eat bigger portions than we need. A study that compared the portions of food offered in the stores and restaurants to the standard serving sizes set

---

FACT BOX 9.2

Is Your Body Mass Index in the Healthy Range?

To find out if your body weight is in the healthy range, you need to do the following:

1) Measure your weight in pounds and your height in inches.

2) Divide your weight by your height, then divide the result by your height again.

3) Multiply the result by 703.

4) If you are 20 years of age or younger, use **Figure 9.1** or **Appendix C** to determine if your BMI is in the healthy range for someone your age.

5) If you are over 20 years of age and your answer falls in the range of 18.5 to 24.9, your BMI is in the healthy range.

by government agencies such as the USDA found that most portions exceed standards by at least a factor of 2 and sometimes 8-fold (Figure 9.2).[32] A third reason for our growing size is that we are burning fewer calories in our daily lives. We ride to work in automobiles rather than walking or biking, we take the elevator instead of the stairs, we use vacuum cleaners rather than brooms, and we often ride our lawn mowers rather than push them. Many schools have reduced or even eliminated physical education programs and in our leisure time we sit in front of televisions, video games, and computers.

Even small changes in the balance between energy intake and energy expenditure could make a big difference in slowing the increase in obesity. It has been estimated that a population-wide shift in energy balance of only 100 calories a day would prevent weight gain in 90% of the population.[33] This means that people would need to eat 100 calories less per day or burn 100 calories more per day or some combination of the two. One hundred calories is the equivalent

---

FACT BOX 9.3

Watch That Serving Size!

On a hot day, a bottle of iced tea or fruit juice may be just what you need to cool off. The label says that a serving has only 100 calories. Take a closer look. The serving size is 8 ounces and the bottle is 20 ounces. So your cool gulp of ice tea may be giving you 250 calories, mostly as added sugars. People tend to eat in units: one cookie, one can, one bottle. You are unlikely to drink half the bottle and save the rest for later. Food manufacturers are required to use standard serving sizes on the label, but they are not required to package products according to these standards. Even if the package is clearly meant to contain multiple servings, you may not always serve yourself the amount listed. For example, if you pour yourself a cup of granola for breakfast, you are probably giving yourself about 4 servings, for a total of over 400 calories. Pasta is also a challenge because the serving size is usually given as dry pasta. What does 2 ounces of spaghetti look like once it is cooked? It looks like about a cup, so if you pile 2 cups onto your plate, you are getting 400 rather than 200 calories with your meal.

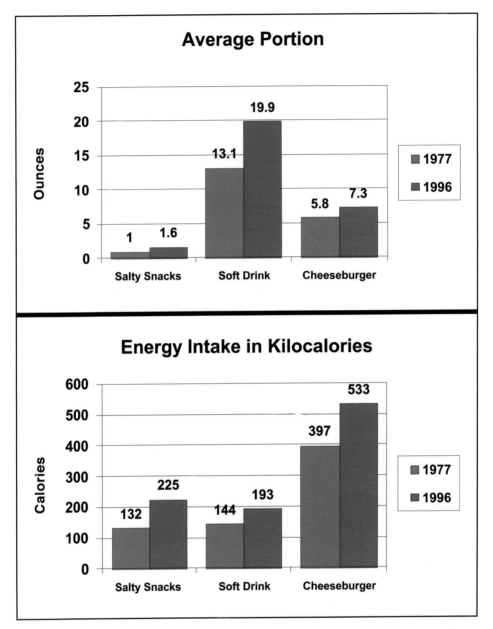

Figure 9.2 The portions of food people eat at home and in restaurants have grown larger since the 1970s, dramatically increasing the number of calories consumed. For example, the average portion of salty snacks has increased 60% since 1977. Soft drink intake has increased nearly that much and the size of a cheeseburger has increased over 25%.

of walking for an extra 15 minutes a day or reducing your ice cream serving to half a cup.

BALANCING CARBOHYDRATE, FAT, AND PROTEIN

You cannot decrease the amount of fat in your diet without increasing the amount of carbohydrate or protein. Likewise, if you cut down on carbohydrates, you will need to increase the amount of fat and protein you eat. Because these nutrients provide the calories you need to stay alive and healthy, if you reduce your intake of one, you need to increase the others to meet your caloric needs. The recommendations of the DRIs recognize this by suggesting ranges of healthy intake: 45% to 60% of calories from carbohydrates, 20% to 35% of our calories as fat, and 10% to 35% of calories as protein (these ranges are for adults and differ slightly for children and adolescents: see Appendix B).[1] Within these ranges, there is no one magic combination of carbohydrate, fat, and protein that results in the optimal diet for everyone. You can choose a pattern that suits your personal preferences and health needs. For example, if you do not eat meat, your dietary pattern will probably be at the high end of the recommended intake for carbohydrates and at the low end of the range for protein. If you prefer a diet high in meat, you may choose one lower in carbohydrates and higher in protein. It is not just the amounts of these nutrients but the types of carbohydrates, fats, and proteins that affect your diet and your health.

Unrefining Your Carbs

A healthy diet not only provides enough carbohydrates to fuel your brain and keep the amounts of protein and fat in a healthy range, but it also includes the right types of carbohydrates. Following the recommendations of the Dietary Guidelines and Food Guide Pyramid can help provide a diet that is based on whole grains, plenty of fruits and vegetables, and limited amounts of added sugars. The key is to choose carbohydrate sources that are less refined. Refining tends to add sugar, salt, and fat, and take out fiber. So fresh blueberries are better than a blueberry pie, fresh tomatoes are better than ketchup, and whole-wheat bread is better than white bread.

The ingredient list on food labels can be helpful in choosing foods that are low in added sugar and high in fiber. Since ingredients are listed in order of their prominence by weight, if a sweetener appears close to the beginning of the list, it is a clue that the food is high in added sugar. Products that list whole wheat or rolled oats as the first ingredient contain mostly these whole grains and are therefore high in fiber. Food labels can be helpful in choosing high-fiber foods because labels are required to list the amount of fiber per serving.

Figuring out Fats

You do not have to eat a diet with only 20% fat to be healthy. A diet with 35% fat can be just as healthy if the types of fat are chosen wisely. The goal is to choose fats that are mono- or polyunsaturated and minimize your consumption of saturated fat, cholesterol, and *trans* fat. Olive oil and canola oils are high in monounsaturated fat; other vegetable oils are high in polyunsaturated fats. Saturated fat and cholesterol are found primarily in animal products such as beef and whole milk. Saturated fat and cholesterol intake can be reduced by choosing reduced fat dairy products and lean meats. *Trans* fat is found in products containing hydrogenated oils, such as solid margarines and shortening. Reducing *trans* fat intake requires limiting these added fats as well as baked goods and other foods that contain them. Soft or liquid margarines and cooking oils are lower in *trans* fats than stick margarine. Fruits, vegetables, and whole grains are naturally cholesterol-free and low in saturated and *trans* fat as long as these fats are not added to them in preparation.

Picking Your Proteins

Most Americans eat plenty of protein. A diet that meets the recommendations of the Food Guide Pyramid provides about 71 grams of protein—more than enough to meet most people's needs. So, which proteins you pick may have more impact on your fat intake than concerns about meeting your protein needs. Animal sources of protein provide high-quality protein, but are often also high in saturated fat and cholesterol. You can enjoy these high-quality proteins without increasing unwanted fats by trimming the fat off your meat and cooking it in ways that do not add fat. For instance, frying food adds fat to it whereas barbecuing allows the fat to drip into the fire instead of into you. Choosing whole grains and legumes to provide some of your protein helps keep your diet low in saturated fat and cholesterol, and high in fiber.

GETTING YOUR VITAMINS

Most foods naturally contain some vitamins and minerals. Cooking, storage, and processing can cause the loss of some of these from foods. Other types of processing can add vitamins and minerals to foods. You can meet your vitamin and mineral needs by choosing a diet that is high in unrefined foods. You can also obtain vitamins and minerals by choosing fortified foods or using vitamin and mineral supplements.

The Benefits of Natural Foods

Food is available in a huge variety of colors and flavors. It also provides a boundless combination of nutrients. Natural food systems are often the best way to meet needs. For instance, dairy foods such as milk and yogurt are good sources of calcium. This calcium comes with the milk sugar lactose that promotes the absorption of calcium. Whole-grain breads are good sources of iron, selenium, zinc, copper, and many B vitamins. When wheat is refined to make the white flour used to bake white bread, much of the iron, selenium, zinc, copper, and B vitamins are lost, but only iron, thiamin, riboflavin, niacin, and folic acid are added when white flour is enriched. Another benefit of obtaining your vitamins and minerals from whole foods is that these foods also provide other health-promoting substances such as phyto-chemicals. Foods high in phytochemicals often provide health benefits that extend beyond basic nutrition. Research studies have repeatedly identified a relationship between diets high in plant foods and thus phytochemicals and a reduction in the incidence of chronic disease.

Fortified Foods

The addition of nutrients to foods is called **fortification**. Some food fortification is mandatory. For example, in the United States, refined grains products must be fortified with the vitamins thiamin, niacin, riboflavin, and folic acid and the mineral iron. Fortification is also a marketing tool used by food manufacturers to make products more appealing to their customers. For example, to increase sales, breakfast cereals are often fortified with so many vitamins that they resemble a multivitamin supplement. Foods fortified with nutrients such as calcium and iron that are low in the American diet can make meeting needs easier for many people. But some foods are fortified with large amounts, so when choosing fortified foods, it is important to be sure your intake does not exceed the UL for any nutrient.

Supplements Can Help or Hurt

Dietary supplements are another source of vitamins and minerals in the American diet. Although most individuals can meet their needs by consuming a varied, balanced diet, individuals who have increased needs, such as pregnant women and children, those whose intake is limited by dietary restrictions, and those whose absorption or utilization is limited by disease may need supplements to meet their needs. Consumers need to be aware, however, that supplements pose a toxicity risk. While it is difficult to consume a toxic amount of a vitamin by eating foods, it is easy to get a large dose in a supplement. Many supplements on the market today also contain substances that are not nutrients, such as herbs. Some of these are safe, but others may have side effects that outweigh any benefits they provide. Because the manufacture of dietary supplements is not strictly regulated and supplements may not be stringently tested for safety before they are marketed, supplements that are dangerous may be on the market for years before enough evidence has accumulated to remove them. If you take supplements, do so with caution.

CONNECTIONS

A healthy diet is one that provides the right number of calories to keep your weight in the healthy range; a balance of carbohydrate, protein, and fat choices; plenty of water; and sufficient but not excessive amounts of essential vitamins and minerals. Maintaining a healthy weight means balancing the calories you consume in your diet with the amount of energy you burn to stay alive and moving. Calorie needs can be estimated using the EER equations. A healthy body weight is a weight that is associated with health and longevity. Unfortunately, many Americans are currently overweight or obese. Many different dietary patterns are healthy, but, in general, a healthy diet should include plenty of unrefined grains, fruits, and vegetables; be limited in saturated fat, *trans* fat, and cholesterol; and provide adequate protein. Vitamin and mineral needs can be met by consuming natural sources of vitamins and minerals as well as by using fortified foods and supplements. The risk of nutrient toxicity is increased when supplements that contain large or imbalanced amounts of nutrients are consumed.

FACT BOX 9.4

How to Choose a Dietary Supplement

Is your supplement safe? Is it providing any benefits? Before you start taking any dietary supplements, ask yourself the following questions:

- Why are you taking the supplement? If you are taking it for insurance, does it provide both vitamins and minerals? If you want to supplement specific nutrients, are they contained in the product?

- Does it contain potentially toxic levels of any nutrient? To find out, check Appendix B to see if the amounts of any nutrients in your supplement exceed the UL.

- Does it contain ingredients other than vitamins and minerals? If so, are these known to be safe?

- Do you have a medical condition that recommends against certain nutrients or other ingredients? If so, be sure your supplement does not contain these.

- Are you taking prescription medication with which the supplement may interact? Check with your physician, dietitian, or pharmacist to help identify these interactions.

- How much does it cost? A high price tag does not always mean it is better. Compare costs and ingredients before you buy.

Appendices

Appendix A

Dietary Reference Intake Values for Energy: Estimated Energy Requirement (EER) Equations and Values for Active Individuals by Life Stage Group

Life Stage Group	EER prediction equation	EER for Active Physical Activity Level (kcal/day)[a]	
		Male	Female
0 – 3 months	EER = (89 x weight of infant in kg – 100) + 175	538	493 (2 mo) [c]
4 – 6 months	EER = (89 x weight of infant in kg – 100) + 56	606	543 (5 mo) [c]
7 – 12 months	EER = (89 x weight of infant in kg – 100) + 22	743	676 (9 mo) [c]
1 – 2 years	EER = (89 x weight of infant in kg – 100) + 20	1046	992 (2 y) [c]
3 – 8 years			
male	EER = 88.5 – (61.9 x Age in yrs) + PA^b[(26.7 x Weight in kg) + (903 x Height in m)] + 20	1742 (6 y)[c]	
female	EER = 135.3 – (30.8 x Age in yrs) + PA^b[(10.0 x Weight in kg) + (934 x Height in m)] + 20		1642 (6 y) [c]
9 – 13 years			
male	EER = 88.5 – (61.9 x Age in yrs) + PA^b [(26.7 x Weight in kg) + (903 x Height in m)] + 25	2279 (11 y) [c]	
female	EER = 135.3 – (30.8 x Age in yrs) + PA^b [(10.0 x Weight in kg) + (934 x Height in m)] + 25		2071 (11 y) [c]
14 – 18 years			
male	EER = 88.5 – (61.9 x Age in yrs) + PA^b [(26.7 x Weight in kg) + (903 x Height in m)] + 25	3152 (16 y) [c]	
female	EER = 135.3 – (30.8 x Age in yrs) + PA^b [(10.0 x Weight in kg) + (934 x Height in m)] + 25		2368 (16 y) [c]
19 and older			
males	EER = 662 – (9.53 x Age in yrs) + PA^b[(15.91 x Weight in kg) + (539.6 x Height in m)]	3067 (19 y) [c]	
females	EER = 354 – (6.91 x Age in yrs) + PA^b[(9.36 x Weight in kg) + (726 x Height in m)]		2403 (19 y) [c]
Pregnancy			
14 –18 years			
1st trimester	Adolescent EER + 0		2368 (16 y) [c]
2nd trimester	Adolescent EER + 340 kcal		2708 (16 y) [c]
3rd trimester	Adolescent EER + 452 kcal		2820 (16 y) [c]
19 – 50 years			
1st trimester	Adult EER + 0		2403 (19 y) [c]
2nd trimester	Adult EER + 340 kcal		2743 (19 y) [c]
3rd trimester	Adult EER + 452 kcal		2855 (19 y) [c]
Lactation			
14 –18 years			
1st 6 mo	Adolescent EER + 330 kcal		2 698 (16 y) [c]
2nd 6 mo	Adolescent EER + 400 kcal		2768 (16 y) [c]
19 – 50 years			
1st 6 mo	Adult EER + 330 kcal		2733 (19 y) [c]
2nd 6 mo	Adult EER + 400 kcal		2803 (19 y) [c]

[a] The intake that meets the average energy expenditure of individuals at a reference height, weight, and age
[b] See table entitled "PA Values" to determine the PA value for various ages, genders, and activity levels
[c] Value is calculated for an individual at the age in parentheses.

PA Values used to calculate EER

Physical Activity Level (PA)	Sedentary	Low active	Active	Very active
3 to 18 years				
Boys	1.00	1.13	1.26	1.42
Girls	1.00	1.16	1.31	1.56
≥ 19 years				
Men	1.00	1.11	1.25	1.48
Women	1.00	1.12	1.27	1.45

Source: Institute of Medicine, Food and Nutrition Board, Dietary Reference Intakes for Energy, Carbohydrates, Fiber, Fat, Protein, and Amino acids. Washington D.C., National Academy Press, 2002.

Acceptable Macronutrient Distribution Ranges (AMDR) for Healthy Diets as a Percent of Energy

Age	Carbohydrate	Added sugars	Total Fat	Linoleic acid	α-Linolenic acid	Protein
1-3 y	45-65	≤25	30-40	5-10	0.6-1.2	5-20
4-18 y	45-65	≤25	25-35	5-10	0.6-1.2	10-30
≥ 19 y	45-65	≤25	20-35	5-10	0.6-1.2	10-35

Source: Institute of Medicine, Food and Nutrition Board. Dietary Reference Intakes for Energy, Carbohydrates, Fiber, Fat, Protein, and Amino Acids. Washington D.C., National Academy Press, 2002.

Dietary Reference Intakes: Recommended Intakes for Individuals: Carbohydrates, Fiber, Fat, Fatty Acids, and Protein

Life Stage Group	Carbohydrate (g/day)	Fiber (g/day)	Fat (g/day)	Linoleic acid (g/day)	α-Linolenic acid (g/day)	Protein (g/kg/day)	Protein (g/day)
Infants							
0-6 mo	60*	ND	31*	4.4*†	0.5*‡	1.52*	9.1*
7-12 mo	95*	ND	30*	4.6*†	0.5*‡	1.5	13.5
Children							
1-3 y	130	19*	ND	7*	0.7*	1.10	13
4-8 y	130	25*	ND	10*	0.9*	0.95	19
Males							
9-13 y	130	31*	ND	12*	1.2*	0.95	34
14-18 y	130	38*	ND	16*	1.6*	0.85	52
19-30 y	130	38*	ND	17*	1.6*	0.80	56
31-50 y	130	38*	ND	17*	1.6*	0.80	56
51-70 y	130	30*	ND	14*	1.6*	0.80	56
> 70 y	130	30*	ND	14*	1.6*	0.80	56
Females							
9-13 y	130	26*	ND	10*	1.0*	0.95	34
14-18 y	130	26*	ND	11*	1.1*	0.85	46
19-30 y	130	25*	ND	12*	1.1*	0.80	46
31-50 y	130	25*	ND	12*	1.1*	0.80	46
51-70 y	130	21*	ND	11*	1.1*	0.80	46
> 70 y	130	21*	ND	11*	1.1*	0.80	46
Pregnancy	175	28*	ND	13*	1.4*	1.1	RDA+25g
Lactation	210	29*	ND	13*	1.3*	1.1	RDA+25g

ND = not determined
* Values are AI (Adequate intakes)
† Refers to all n-6 polyunsaturated fatty acids
‡ Refers to all n-3 polyunsaturated fatty acids

Source: Institute of Medicine, Food and Nutrition Board, Dietary Reference Intakes for Energy, Carbohydrates, Fiber, Fat, Protein, and Amino Acids. Washington D.C., National Academy Press, 2002.

Appendix B

Dietary Reference Intakes: Recommened Intakes for Individuals: Vitamins

Life Stage Group	Vitamin A (µg/day)[a]	Vitamin C (mg/day)	Vitamin D (µg/day)[b,c]	Vitamin E (mg/day)[d]	Vitamin K (µg/day)	Thiamin (mg/day)	Riboflavin (mg/day)	Niacin (mg/day)[e]	Vitamin B_6 (mg/day)	Folate (µg/day)[f]	Vitamin B_{12} (µg/day)	Pantothenic Acid (mg/day)	Biotin (µg/day)	Choline[g] (mg/day)
Infants														
0-6 mo	400*	40*	5*	4*	2.0*	0.2*	0.3*	2*	0.1*	65*	0.4*	1.7*	5*	125*
7-12 mo	500*	50*	5*	5*	2.5*	0.3*	0.4*	4*	0.3*	80*	0.5*	1.8*	6*	150*
Children														
1-3 y	**300**	**15**	5*	**6**	30*	**0.5**	**0.5**	**6**	**0.5**	**150**	**0.9**	2*	8*	200*
4-8 y	**400**	**25**	5*	**7**	55*	**0.6**	**0.6**	**8**	**0.5**	**200**	**1.2**	3*	12*	250*
Males														
9-13 y	**600**	**45**	5*	**11**	60*	**0.9**	**0.9**	**12**	**1.0**	**300**	**1.8**	4*	20*	375*
14-18 y	**900**	**75**	5*	**15**	75*	**1.2**	**1.3**	**16**	**1.3**	**400**	**2.4**	5*	25*	550*
19-30 y	**900**	**90**	5*	**15**	120*	**1.2**	**1.3**	**16**	**1.3**	**400**	**2.4**	5*	30*	550*
31-50 y	**900**	**90**	5*	**15**	120*	**1.2**	**1.3**	**16**	**1.3**	**400**	**2.4**	5*	30*	550*
51-70 y	**900**	**90**	10*	**15**	120*	**1.2**	**1.3**	**16**	**1.7**	**400**	**2.4**[h]	5*	30*	550*
> 70 y	**900**	**90**	15*	**15**	120*	**1.2**	**1.3**	**16**	**1.7**	**400**	**2.4**[h]	5*	30*	550*
Females														
9-13 y	**600**	**45**	5*	**11**	60*	**0.9**	**0.9**	**12**	**1.0**	**300**	**1.8**	4*	20*	375*
14-18 y	**700**	**65**	5*	**15**	75*	**1.0**	**1.0**	**14**	**1.2**	**400**[i]	**2.4**	5*	25*	400*
19-30 y	**700**	**75**	5*	**15**	90*	**1.1**	**1.1**	**14**	**1.3**	**400**[i]	**2.4**	5*	30*	425*
31-50 y	**700**	**75**	5*	**15**	90*	**1.1**	**1.1**	**14**	**1.3**	**400**[i]	**2.4**	5*	30*	425*
51-70 y	**700**	**75**	10*	**15**	90*	**1.1**	**1.1**	**14**	**1.5**	**400**	**2.4**[h]	5*	30*	425*
> 70 y	**700**	**75**	15*	**15**	90*	**1.1**	**1.1**	**14**	**1.5**	**400**	**2.4**[h]	5*	30*	425*
Pregnancy														
≤ 18 y	**750**	**80**	5*	**15**	75*	**1.4**	**1.4**	**18**	**1.9**	**600**[j]	**2.6**	6*	30*	450*
14-18 y	**770**	**85**	5*	**15**	90*	**1.4**	**1.4**	**18**	**1.9**	**600**[j]	**2.6**	6*	30*	450*
19-30 y	**770**	**85**	5*	**15**	90*	**1.4**	**1.4**	**18**	**1.9**	**600**[j]	**2.6**	6*	30*	450*
Lactation														
≤ 18 y	**1200**	**115**	5*	**19**	75*	**1.4**	**1.6**	**17**	**2.0**	**500**	**2.8**	7*	35*	550*
14-18 y	**1300**	**120**	5*	**19**	90*	**1.4**	**1.6**	**17**	**2.0**	**500**	**2.8**	7*	35*	550*
19-30 y	**1300**	**120**	5*	**19**	90*	**1.4**	**1.6**	**17**	**2.0**	**500**	**2.8**	7*	35*	550*

NOTE: This table (taken from the DRI reports, see www.nap.edu) presents Recommended Dietary Allowances (RDAs) in **bold** type and Adequate Intakes (AIs) in ordinary type followed by an asterisk (*). RDAs and AIs may both be used as goals for individual intakes. RDAs are set up to meet the needs of almost all (97–98%) individuals in a group. For healthy breastfed infants, the AI is the mean intake. The AI for all other life stage and gender groups is believed to cover needs of all individuals in the group, but lack of data or uncertainty in the data prevent being able to specify with confidence the percentage of individuals covered by this intake.

[a]As retinol activity equivalents (RAEs). 1 RAE = 1 µg retinol, 12 µg β-carotene, 24 µg β-carotene, or 24 µg β-cryptoxanthin in foods. TO calculate RAEs from REs of provitamin A carotenoids in foods, divide RE by 2. For preformed vitamin A in foods or supplements and for provitamin A carotenoids in supplements, 1 RE = 1 RAE.

[b]Cholecalciferol. 1 µg cholecalciferol = 40 IU vitamin D.

[c]In the absence of exposure to adequate sunlight.

[d]As α-tocopherol, which includes RRR-α-tocopherol, the only form of α-tocopherol that occurs naturally in foods, and the 2R-stereoisomeric forms of α-tocopherol (RRR-, RSR-, RRS-, and RSS-α-tocopherol). Does not include the 2S-stereoisomeric forms of α-tocopherol (SRR-, SSR-, SRS-, and SSS- α -tocopherol), also found in food and supplements.

[e]As niacin equivalents (NEs), 1mg niacin = 60 mg tryptophan; 0-6 months = preformed niacin (not NE).

[f]As dietary folate equivalents (DFEs). 1 DFE = 1 µg food folate = 0.6 µg folic acid from fortified food or as a supplement consumed with food = 0.5 µg of a supplement taken on an empty stomach.

[g]Although AIs have been set for choline, there are few data to assess whether a dietary supplement of choline is needed at all stages of the lifecycle, and it may be that the choline requirement can be met by endogenous synthesis at some of these stages.

[h]Because 10-30% of older people may malabsorb food-bound B_{12}, it is advisable for those older than 50 years to meet their RFD mainly by consuming foods fortified with B_{12} or containing B_{12}.

[i]In view of evidence linking folate intake with neural tube defects in the fetus, it is recommended that all women capable of becoming pregnant consume 400 µg from supplements or fortified foods in addition to intake of food folate from a varied diet.

[j]It is assumed that women will consume 400 µg from supplements or fortified foods until their pregnancy is confirmed and they enter prenatal care, which ordinarily occurs after the end of the periconceptional period – the critical time for neural tube formation.

Source: Trumbo, P., A. Yates, S. Schlicker, M. Poos. "Dietary Reference Intakes: Vitamin A, Vitamin K, Arsenic, Boron, Chrominm, Copper, Iodine, Iron, Manganese, Molybdenum, Nickel, Silicon, Vanadium, and Zinc." *Journal of the American Dietetic Association* 101, no. 3 (2001) 294-301.

Dietary Reference Intakes: Recommended Intakes for Individuals: Minerals

Life Stage Group	Calcium (mg/day)	Chromium (µg/day)	Copper (µg/day)	Fluoride (mg/day)	Iodine (µg/day)	Iron (mg/day)	Magnesium (mg/day)	Manganese (mg/day)	Molybdenum (µg/day)	Phosphorus (mg/day)	Selenium (µg/day)	Zinc (mg/day)
Infants												
0-6 mo	210*	0.2*	200*	0.01*	110*	0.27*	30*	0.003*	2*	100*	15*	2*
7-12 mo	270*	5.5*	220*	0.5*	130*	11	75*	0.6*	3*	275*	20*	3
Children												
1-3 y	500*	11*	340	0.7*	90	7	80	1.2*	17	460	20	3
4-8 y	800*	15*	440	1*	90	10	130	1.5*	22	500	30	5
Males												
9-13 y	1,300*	25*	700	2*	120	8	240	1.9*	34	1,250	40	8
14-18 y	1,300*	35*	890	3*	150	11	410	2.2*	43	1,250	55	11
19-30 y	1,000*	35*	900	4*	150	8	400	2.3*	45	700	55	11
31-50 y	1,000*	35*	900	4*	150	8	420	2.3*	45	700	55	11
51-70 y	1,200*	30*	900	4*	150	8	420	2.3*	45	700	55	11
>70 y	1,200*	30*	900	4*	150	8	420	2.3*	45	700	55	11
Females												
9-13 y	1,300*	21*	700	2*	120	8	240	1.6*	34	1,250	40	8
14-18 y	1,300*	24*	890	3*	150	15	360	1.6*	43	1,250	55	9
19-30 y	1,000*	25*	900	3*	150	18	310	1.8*	45	700	55	8
31-50 y	1,000*	25*	900	3*	150	18	320	1.8*	45	700	55	8
51-70 y	1,200*	20*	900	3*	150	8	320	1.8*	45	700	55	8
>70 y	1,200*	20*	900	3*	150	8	320	1.8*	45	700	55	8
Pregnancy												
≤18 y	1,300*	29*	1,000	3*	220	27	400	2.0*	50	1,250	60	13
14-18 y	1,000*	30*	1,000	3*	220	27	350	2.0*	50	700	60	11
19-30 y	1,000*	30*	1,000	3*	220	27	360	2.0*	50	700	60	11
Lactation												
≤18 y	1,300*	44*	1,300	3*	290	10	360	2.6*	50	1,250	70	14
14-18 y	1,300*	45*	1,300	3*	290	9	310	2.6*	50	700	70	12
19-30 y	1,300*	45*	1,300	3*	290	9	320	2.6*	50	700	70	12

NOTE: This table (taken from the DRI reports, see www.nap.edu) presents Recommended Dietary Allowances (RDAs) in **bold** type and Adequate Intakes (AIs) in ordinary type followed by an asterisk (*). RDAs and AIs may both be used as goals for individual intakes. RDAs are set up to meet the needs of almost all (97-98%) individuals in a group. For healthy breastfed infants, the AI is the mean intake. The AI for all other life stage and gender groups is believed to cover needs of all individuals in the group, but lack of data or uncertainty in the data prevent being able to specify with confidence the percentage of individuals covered by this intake.

151

Appendix B

Dietary Reference Intakes (DRIs): Tolerable Upper Intake Levels (UL[a]): Vitamins

Life Stage Group	Vitamin A (μg/day)[b]	Vitamin C (mg/day)	Vitamin D (μg/day)	Vitamin E (mg/day)[c,d]	Vitamin K	Thiamin	Riboflavin	Niacin (mg/day)[d]	Vitamin B6 (mg/day)	Folate (μg/day)[d]	Vitamin B12	Pantothenic Acid	Biotin	Choline (mg/day)	Carotenoids[e]
Infants															
0-6 mo	600	ND[f]	25	ND[f]	ND	ND	ND	ND	ND	ND	ND	ND	ND	ND	ND
7-12 mo	600	ND	25	ND	ND	ND	ND	ND	ND	ND	ND	ND	ND	ND	ND
Children															
1-3 y	600	400	50	200	ND	ND	ND	10	30	300	ND	ND	ND	1.0	ND
4-8 y	900	650	50	300	ND	ND	ND	15	40	400	ND	ND	ND	1.0	ND
Males, Females															
9-13 y	1,700	1,200	50	600	ND	ND	ND	20	60	600	ND	ND	ND	2.0	ND
14-18 y	2,800	1,800	50	800	ND	ND	ND	30	80	800	ND	ND	ND	3.0	ND
19-70 y	3,000	2,000	50	1,000	ND	ND	ND	35	100	1,000	ND	ND	ND	3.5	ND
>70 y	3,000	2,000	50	1,000	ND	ND	ND	35	100	1,000	ND	ND	ND	3.5	ND
Pregnancy															
≤18 y	2,800	1,800	50	800	ND	ND	ND	30	80	800	ND	ND	ND	3.0	ND
19-50 y	3,000	2,000	50	1,000	ND	ND	ND	35	100	1,000	ND	ND	ND	3.5	ND
Lactation															
≤18 y	2,800	1,800	50	800	ND	ND	ND	30	80	800	ND	ND	ND	3.0	ND
19-50 y	3,000	2,000	50	1,000	ND	ND	ND	35	100	1,000	ND	ND	ND	3.5	ND

[a]UL = The maximum level of daily nutrient intake that is likely to pose no risk of adverse effects. Unless otherwise specified, the UL represents total intake from food, water, and supplements. Due to lack of suitable data, ULs could not be established for vitamin K, thiamin, riboflavin, vitamin B12, pantothenic acid, biotin, or carotenoids. In the absence of ULs, extra caution may be warranted in consuming levels above recommended intakes.

[b]As preformed vitamin A only.

[c]As α-tocopherol; applies to any for of supplemental α-tocopherol.

[d]The ULs for vitamin E, niacin, and folate apply to synthetic forms obtained from supplements, fortified foods, or a combination of the two.

[e]β-Carotene supplements are advised only to serve as a provitamin A source for individuals at risk of vitamin A deficiency.

[f]ND=Not determinable due to lack of data of adverse effects in this age group and concern with regard to lack of ability to handle excess amounts. Source of intakes should be from food only to prevent high levels of intake.

152

Dietary Reference Intakes (DRIs): Tolerable Upper Intake Levels (UL[a]): Minerals

Life Stage Group	Arsenic[b]	Boron (mg/day)	Calcium (g/day)	Chromium	Copper (µg/day)	Fluoride (mg/day)	Iodine (µg/day)	Iron (mg/day)	Magnesium (mg/day)[c]	Manganese (mg/day)	Molybdenum (µg/day)	Nickel (mg/day)	Phosphorus (g/day)	Selenium (µg/day)	Silicon[d]	Vanadium (mg/day)[e]	Zinc (mg/day)
Infants																	
0-6 mo	ND[f]	ND	ND	ND	ND	0.7	ND	40	ND	ND	ND	ND	ND	45	ND	ND	4
7-12 mo	ND	ND	ND	ND	ND	0.9	ND	40	ND	ND	ND	ND	ND	60	ND	ND	5
Children																	
1-3 y	ND	3	2.5	ND	1,000	1.3	200	40	65	2	300	0.2	3	90	ND	ND	7
4-8 y	ND	6	2.5	ND	3,000	2.2	300	40	110	3	600	0.3	3	150	ND	ND	12
Males, Females																	
9-13 y	ND	11	2.5	ND	5,000	10	600	40	350	6	1,100	0.6	4	280	ND	ND	23
14-18 y	ND	17	2.5	ND	8,000	10	900	45	350	9	1,700	1.0	4	400	ND	ND	34
19-70 y	ND	20	2.5	ND	10,000	10	1,100	45	350	11	2,000	1.0	4	400	ND	1.8	40
>70 y	ND	20	2.5	ND	10,000	10	1,100	45	350	11	2,000	1.0	3	400	ND	1.8	40
Pregnancy																	
≤18 y	ND	17	2.5	ND	8,000	10	900	45	350	9	1,700	1.0	3.5	400	ND	ND	34
19-50 y	ND	20	2.5	ND	10,000	10	1,100	45	350	11	2,000	1.0	3.5	400	ND	ND	40
Lactation																	
≤18 y	ND	17	2.5	ND	8,000	10	900	45	350	9	1,700	1.0	4	400	ND	ND	34
19-50 y	ND	20	2.5	ND	10,000	10	1,100	45	350	11	2,000	1.0	4	400	ND	ND	40

[a]UL= the maximum level of daily nutrient intake that is likely to pose no risk of adverse effects. Unless otherwise specified, the UL represents total intake from food, water, and supplements. Due to lack of suitable data, ULs could not be established for arsenic, chromium, and silicon. In the absence of ULs, extra cautopm may be warranted in consuming levels above recommended intakes.

[b]Although the UL was not determined for arsenic, there is no justification for adding arsenic to food or supplements.

[c]The ULs for magnesium represent intake from a pharmacological agent only and do not include intake from food and water.

[d]Although silicon has not been shown to cause adverse effects in humans, there is no justification for adding silicon to supplements.

[e]Although vanadium in food has not been shown to cause adverse effects in humans, there is no justification for adding vanadium to food and vanadium supplements should be used with caution is based on adverse effects in laboratory animals and this data could be used to set a UL for adults from not children and adolescents.

[f]ND=Not determinable due to lack of data of adverse effects in this age group and concern with regard to lack of ability to handle excess amunts. Source of intake should be from food only to prev\ levels of intake.

153

Dietary Reference Intakes: Recommended Intakes and Tolerable Upper Intake Levels (UL): Water, Potassium, Sodium, and Chloride						
Life Stage Group	Water[a] (liters)	Potassium[a,b] (mg)	Sodium (mg)		Chloride (mg)	
			Recommended Intake	UL	Recommended Intake	UL
Infants						
0–6 mo	0.7	0.4	0.12	-	0.18	-
7–12 mo	0.8	0.7	0.37	-	0.58	-
Children						
1–3 y	1.3	3.0	1.0	1.5	1.5	2.3
4–8 y	1.7	3.8	1.2	1.9	1.9	2.9
Males						
9–13 y	2.4	4.5	1.5	2.2	2.3	3.4
14–18 y	3.3	4.7	1.5	2.3	2.3	3.6
19–30 y	3.7	4.7	1.5	2.3	2.3	3.6
31–50 y	3.7	4.7	1.5	2.3	2.3	3.6
51–70 y	3.7	4.7	1.3	2.3	2.0	3.6
>70 y	3.7	4.7	1.2	2.3	1.8	3.6
Females						
9–13 y	2.1	4.5	1.5	2.2	2.3	3.4
14–18 y	2.3	4.7	1.5	2.3	2.3	3.6
19–30 y	2.7	4.7	1.5	2.3	2.3	3.6
31–50 y	2.7	4.7	1.5	2.3	2.3	3.6
51–70 y	2.7	4.7	1.3	2.3	2.0	3.6
>70 y	2.7	4.7	1.2	2.3	1.8	3.6

[a] No UL has been established for water or potassium.
[b] The recommended intake is the same for all groups over 14 years except lactating women = 5.1 mg

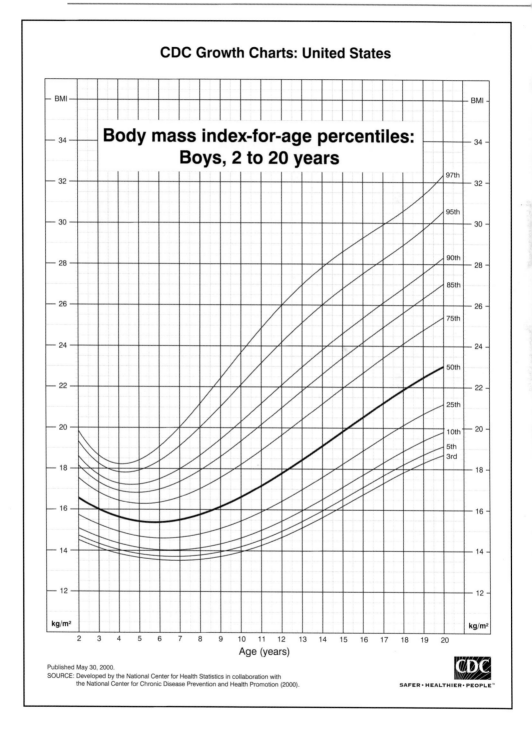

CDC Growth Charts: United States

Body mass index-for-age percentiles: Boys, 2 to 20 years

Published May 30, 2000.
SOURCE: Developed by the National Center for Health Statistics in collaboration with the National Center for Chronic Disease Prevention and Health Promotion (2000).

CDC
SAFER · HEALTHIER · PEOPLE™

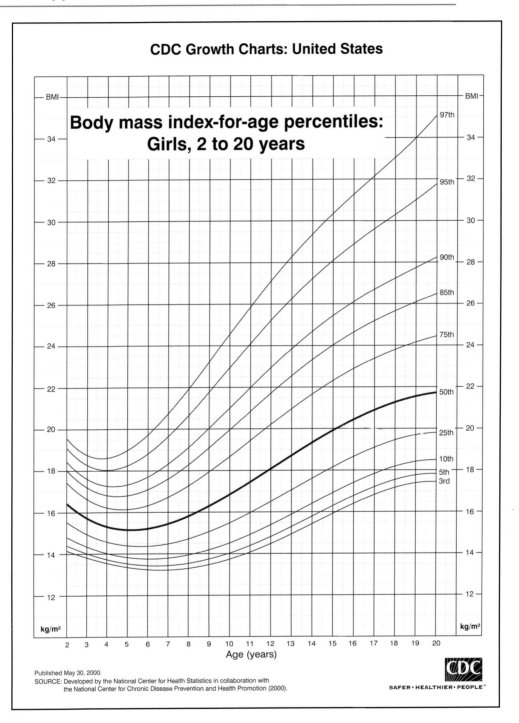

CDC Growth Charts: United States

Body mass index-for-age percentiles: Girls, 2 to 20 years

Published May 30, 2000.
SOURCE: Developed by the National Center for Health Statistics in collaboration with the National Center for Chronic Disease Prevention and Health Promotion (2000).

Glossary

Absorption The process of taking substances into the body.

Adenosine triphosphate (ATP) The high-energy molecule used by the body to perform energy-requiring activities.

Adequate Intakes (AIs) Intakes recommended by the DRIs that should be used as a goal when no RDA exists. These values are an approximation of the average nutrient intake that appears to sustain a desired indicator of health.

Adipose tissue Tissue found under the skin and around body organs that is composed of fat-storing cells.

Aerobic Occurring in the presence of oxygen.

Aldosterone A hormone that increases sodium reabsorption and therefore enhances water retention by the kidney.

Alpha-tocopherol (α-tocopherol) The only form of tocopherol that provides vitamin E activity in humans.

Amino acids The building blocks of proteins. Each contains a carbon atom bound to a hydrogen atom, an amino group, an acid group, and a side chain.

Amylase An enzyme secreted by the salivary glands that breaks down starch.

Anabolic steroids Synthetic fat-soluble hormones used by some athletes to increase muscle mass.

Anaerobic Occurring in the absence of oxygen.

Angiotensin II A compound that causes blood vessel walls to constrict and stimulates the release of the hormone aldosterone.

Antibodies Proteins produced by cells of the immune system that destroy or deactivate foreign substances in the body.

Anticoagulant A substance that delays or prevents blood clotting.

Antidiuretic hormone (ADH) A hormone secreted by the pituitary gland that increases the amount of water reabsorbed by the kidney and therefore retained in the body.

Antioxidant A substance that is able to neutralize reactive molecules and hence reduce the amount of oxidative damage that occurs.

Ariboflavinosis A deficiency of the vitamin riboflavin.

Arteries Vessels that carry blood away from the heart.

Ascorbate or **Ascorbic acid** The chemical term for vitamin C.

Atherosclerosis A type of cardiovascular disease that involves the buildup of fatty material in the artery walls.

ATP See adenosine triphosphate.

Beriberi The disease resulting from a deficiency of thiamin.

Beta-carotene (β-carotene) A carotenoid that has more provitamin A activity than other carotenoids. It also acts as an antioxidant.

Bile A substance made in the liver and stored in the gallbladder. It is released into the small intestine to aid in fat digestion and absorption.

Bile acids Emulsifiers present in bile that are synthesized by the liver from cholesterol.

Bioavailability A general term that refers to how well a nutrient can be absorbed and used by the body.

Blood pressure The amount of force exerted by the blood against the artery walls.

BMI (Body Mass Index) The current standard for assessing body weight. A BMI between 18.5 and 24.9 is considered healthy for adults.

Bran The protective outer layers of whole grains. It is a concentrated source of dietary fiber.

Buffer A substance that reacts with an acid or base by picking up or releasing hydrogen ions to prevent changes in pH.

Calcitonin A hormone secreted by the thyroid gland that reduces blood calcium levels.

Calorie The amount of heat needed to raise the temperature of one gram of water by 1°C. It is commonly used to refer to a kilocalorie, which is 1,000 calories.

Glossary

Capillaries Small, thin-walled blood vessels where the exchange of gases and nutrients between blood and cells occurs.

Carbohydrate loading or **glycogen supercompensation** A regimen of diet and exercise that is designed to load muscle glycogen stores beyond their normal capacity.

Cardiovascular disease Any disease affecting the heart and blood vessels.

Carotenoids Natural pigments synthesized by plants and many microorganisms. They give yellow and red-orange fruits and vegetables their color.

Cell differentiation Structural and functional changes that cause cells to mature into specialized cells.

Cell membrane The membrane that surrounds the cell contents.

Cells The basic structural and functional units of plant and animal life.

Cellular respiration The reactions that break down glucose, fatty acids, and amino acids in the presence of oxygen to produce carbon dioxide, water, and energy in the form of ATP.

Ceruloplasmin A copper-containing protein that converts iron to the ferric form, which can bind to iron storage and iron transport proteins.

Chemical bonds Forces that hold atoms together.

Cholecalciferol The chemical name for vitamin D_3. It can be formed in the skin of animals by the action of sunlight on a form of cholesterol called 7-dehydrocholesterol.

Cholesterol A lipid made only by animal cells that consists of multiple chemical rings.

Chylomicrons Lipoproteins that transport lipids from the mucosal cells of the intestine to other body cells.

Citric acid cycle Also known as the Krebs cycle or the tricarboxylic acid cycle, this is the stage of respiration in which acetyl CoA is broken down into 2 molecules of carbon dioxide.

Cobalamin The chemical term for vitamin B_{12}.

Coenzymes Small nonprotein organic molecules that act as carriers of electrons or atoms in metabolic reactions and are necessary for the proper functioning of many enzymes.

Cofactor A mineral or a coenzyme required for enzyme activity.

Collagen The major protein in connective tissue.

Colon The largest portion of the large intestine.

Complex carbohydrates Carbohydrates composed of sugar molecules linked together in straight or branching chains. They include starches and fibers.

Cretinism A condition resulting from poor maternal iodine intake during pregnancy that causes stunted growth and poor mental development in offspring.

Cytoplasm The cellular material outside the nucleus that is contained by the cell membrane.

Daily Value A nutrient reference value used on food labels to help consumers see how foods fit into their overall diets.

DASH diet A dietary pattern that lowers blood pressure. It is high in fruits, vegetables, and low-fat dairy products and therefore high in potassium, magnesium, calcium, and fiber, and low in saturated fat and cholesterol.

Dental caries The decay and deterioration of teeth caused by acid produced when bacteria on the teeth metabolize carbohydrates.

Diabetes or diabetes mellitus A disease caused by either insufficient insulin production or decreased sensitivity of cells to insulin. It results in elevated blood glucose levels.

Dietary References Intakes (DRIs) A set of reference values for the intake of nutrients and food components that can be used for planning and assessing the diets of healthy people in the United States and Canada.

Digestion The process of breaking food into components small enough to be absorbed into the body.

Disaccharide A sugar formed by linking two monosaccharides.

Glossary

Diverticulosis A condition in which sacs or pouches form in the wall of the large intestine. When these become inflamed, the condition is called diverticulitis.

Eicosanoids Regulatory molecules that can be synthesized from omega-3 and omega-6 fatty acids.

Electrolytes Substances that form positively and negatively charged ions when dissolved in water. In nutrition this term refers to sodium, potassium, and chloride.

Electron transport chain The final stage of cellular respiration in which electrons are passed down a chain of molecules to oxygen to form water and produce ATP.

Elements Substances that cannot be broken down into products with different properties.

Empty calories Refers to foods that contribute energy but few nutrients.

Emulsifiers Substances that allow water and fat to mix.

Endosperm The largest portion of a kernel of grain. It is primarily starch and serves as a food supply for the sprouting seed.

Enrichment A term used to describe the addition of nutrients to a food in order to restore those lost in processing to a level equal to or higher than that originally present.

Enzymes Protein molecules that accelerate the rate of specific chemical reactions without being changed themselves.

Esophagus A portion of the gastrointestinal tract that extends from the throat to the stomach.

Essential fatty acid deficiency A condition characterized by dry, scaly skin and poor growth that results when the diet does not supply sufficient amounts of the essential fatty acids.

Essential or indispensable amino acids Amino acids that cannot be synthesized by the human body in sufficient amounts to meet needs and therefore must be included in the diet.

Essential nutrients Nutrients that must be supplied in the diet because they cannot be made in sufficient quantities in the body to meet needs.

Estimated Average Requirements (EARs) Intakes recommended by the DRIs that meet the estimated nutrient needs of 50% of individuals in a gender and life-stage group.

Estimated Energy Requirements (EERs) Energy intakes recommended by the DRIs to maintain body weight.

Extracellular fluid The fluid located outside cells. It includes fluid found in the blood, lymph, gastrointestinal tract, spinal column, eyes, and joints, and that found between cells and tissues.

Fat-soluble vitamins Vitamins that dissolve in fat.

Fatty acid An organic molecule made up of a chain of carbons linked to hydrogens with an acid group at one end.

Feces Body waste, including unabsorbed food residue, bacteria, mucus, and dead cells, which is excreted from the gastrointestinal tract by passing through the anus.

Ferritin The major iron storage protein.

Fiber Nonstarch polysaccharides in plant foods that are not broken down by human digestive enzymes.

Fortification A term used generally to describe the addition of nutrients to foods, such as the addition of vitamin D to milk.

Free radical One type of highly reactive molecule that causes oxidative damage.

Fructose A monosaccharide that is sweeter to the taste than glucose.

Galactose A monosaccharide that along with glucose makes up lactose.

Gallbladder An organ of the digestive system that stores bile, which is produced by the liver.

Gastrointestinal tract A hollow tube consisting of the mouth, pharynx, esophagus, stomach, small intestine, large intestine, and anus, in which digestion and absorption of nutrients occurs.

Gene A section of DNA that codes for a protein.

Gene expression Refers to the events of protein synthesis in which the information coded in a gene is used to synthesize a protein.

Glossary

Germ The embryo or sprouting portion of a kernel of grain. It contains vegetable oil and vitamins.

Glucagon A hormone made in the pancreas that stimulates the breakdown of liver glycogen and the synthesis of glucose to increase blood sugar.

Gluconeogenesis The synthesis of glucose from simple noncarbohydrate molecules. Amino acids from protein are the primary source of carbons for glucose synthesis.

Glucose A monosaccharide that is the primary form of carbohydrate used to produce energy in the body. It is the sugar referred to as blood sugar.

Glycogen A carbohydrate made of many glucose molecules linked together in a highly branched structure. It is the storage form of carbohydrate in animals.

Glycogen supercompensation A regimen of diet and exercise that is designed to load muscle glycogen stores beyond their normal capacity. Also known as carbohydrate loading.

Glycolysis A metabolic pathway in the cytoplasm of the cell that splits glucose into two 3-carbon pyruvate molecules. The energy released from 1 molecule of glucose is used to make 2 ATP molecules.

Goiter An enlargement of the thyroid gland caused by a deficiency of iodine.

Heme iron A readily absorbed form of iron found in animal products that is chemically associated with proteins such as hemoglobin and myoglobin.

Hemochromatosis An inherited condition that results in increased iron absorption.

Hemoglobin An iron-containing protein in red blood cells that binds and transports oxygen through the bloodstream to cells.

High-density lipoproteins (HDLs) Lipoproteins that pick up cholesterol from cells and transport it to the liver so that it can be eliminated from the body. A low level of HDL increases the risk of cardio-vascular disease.

Homeostasis A physiological state in which a stable internal body environment is maintained.

Homocysteine An intermediate in the metabolism of methionine. High levels in the blood increase the risk of heart disease.

Hormones Chemical messengers that are produced in one location, released into the blood, and that elicit responses at other locations in the body.

Hydrogenation The process whereby hydrogens are added to the carbon-carbon double bonds of unsaturated fatty acids, making them more saturated.

Hypercarotenemia A condition caused by an accumulation of carotenoids in the adipose tissue, causing the skin to appear yellow-orange.

Hypertension Blood pressure that is consistently elevated to 140/90 mm of mercury or greater.

Hyponatremia A relative insufficiency of sodium such that the concentration of sodium in body fluids is reduced.

Inorganic Containing no carbon atoms.

Insensible losses Fluid losses that are not perceived by the senses, such as evaporation of water through the skin and lungs.

Insoluble fiber Fiber that, for the most part, does not dissolve in water. It includes cellulose, hemicelluloses, and lignin.

Insulin A hormone made in the pancreas that allows the uptake of glucose by body cells and has other metabolic effects such as stimulating the synthesis of glycogen in liver and muscle.

Interstitial fluid The portion of the extracellular fluid located in the spaces between cells and tissues.

Intestinal microflora Microorganisms that inhabit the large intestine.

Intracellular fluid The fluid located inside cells.

Intrinsic factor A protein produced in the stomach that is needed for the absorption of adequate amounts of vitamin B_{12}.

Ion An atom or group of atoms that carries a negative or a positive electrical charge.

Glossary

Iron deficiency anemia A condition that occurs when the oxygen-carrying capacity of the blood is decreased because there is insufficient iron to make hemoglobin.

Keratin A hard protein that makes up hair and nails.

Ketones or **ketone bodies** Molecules formed when there is not sufficient carbohydrate to completely metabolize the acetyl CoA produced from fat breakdown.

Kilocalorie A unit of heat that is used to express the amount of energy provided by foods.

Kilojoule A measure of work that can be used to express energy intake and energy output; 4.18 kjoules = 1 kcalorie.

Kwashiorkor A form of protein-energy malnutrition in which only protein is deficient. It is most common in young children who are unable to meet their high protein needs with the available diet.

Lactic acid An acid produced from pyruvate in the absence of oxygen that can build up in muscles and contribute to fatigue.

Lactose The disaccharide comprised of glucose and galactose. It is the sugar found in milk and other dairy products.

Lactose intolerance The inability to digest lactose because of a deficiency of the enzyme lactase. It causes symptoms including intestinal gas and bloating after dairy products are consumed.

Lecithin A phosphoglyceride that is a major component of cell membranes and is used as an emulsifier in foods.

Limiting amino acid The amino acid in shortest supply in relation to need.

Lipases Fat-digesting enzymes.

Lipid A group of organic molecules, most of which do not dissolve in water. They include fatty acids, glycerides, phospholipids, and sterols.

Lipid bilayer Two layers of phosphoglyceride molecules oriented so that the fat-soluble fatty acid tails are sandwiched between the water-soluble phosphate-containing heads.

Lipoproteins Particles containing a core of lipids surrounded by a shell of protein and phospholipid that transport lipids in blood and lymph.

Low-density lipoproteins (LDLs) Lipoproteins that transport cholesterol to cells. Elevated LDL cholesterol increases the risk of cardiovascular disease.

Lumen The inside cavity of a tube, such as the gastrointestinal tract.

Lymphatic system The system of vessels, organs, and tissues that drains excess fluid from the spaces between cells, picks up fat-soluble substances absorbed from the digestive tract, and provides immune function.

Macrocytic or **megaloblastic anemia** A condition in which there are abnormally large immature and mature red blood cells and a reduction in the total number of red blood cells.

Macronutrients Nutrients needed by the body in large amounts. These include water and the energy-yielding nutrients carbohydrates, lipids, and proteins.

Major minerals Minerals needed in the diet in amounts greater than 100 mg per day or present in the body in amounts greater than 0.01% of body weight.

Malnutrition Any condition resulting from an energy or nutrient intake either above or below that which is optimal.

Maltose A disaccharide consisting of two molecules of glucose.

Marasmus A form of protein-energy malnutrition in which a deficiency of energy in the diet causes severe body wasting.

Menaquinones The forms of vitamin K synthesized by bacteria and found in animals.

Metabolism The sum of all the chemical reactions that take place in a living organism.

Micronutrients Nutrients needed by the body in small amounts. These include vitamins and minerals.

Mitochondria The cellular organelle responsible for generating energy in the form of ATP for cellular activities.

Glossary

Molecules Units of two or more atoms of the same or different elements bonded together.

Monosaccharide A single sugar molecule, such as glucose.

Monounsaturated fatty acid A fatty acid that contains one carbon-carbon double bond.

Mucus A viscous fluid secreted by glands in the gastrointestinal tract and other parts of the body. It acts to lubricate, moisten, and protect cells from harsh environments.

Myoglobin An iron-containing protein in muscle cells.

Neural tube defects Abnormalities in the brain or spinal cord that result from errors that occur during prenatal development.

Neurotransmitter A chemical substance produced by a nerve cell that can stimulate or inhibit another cell.

Nonheme iron A poorly absorbed form of iron found in both plant and animal foods that is not part of the iron complex found in hemoglobin and myoglobin.

Nutrient density A measure of the nutrients provided by a food relative to the energy it contains.

Nutrients Chemical substances in foods that provide energy, structure, and regulation for body processes.

Nutrition A science that studies the interactions that occur between living organisms and food.

Oligosaccharides Short chain carbohydrates containing 3 to 10 sugar units.

Omega-6 (ω6) fatty acid A fatty acid containing a carbon-carbon double bond between the sixth and seventh carbons from the omega end.

Omega-3 (ω3) fatty acid A fatty acid containing a carbon-carbon double bond between the third and fourth carbons from the omega end.

Organic Molecules that contain two or more carbon atoms.

Osmosis The passive movement of water across a membrane to equalize the concentration of dissolved solutes on both sides.

Osteomalacia A vitamin D deficiency disease in adults characterized by loss of minerals from the bone matrix. It causes weak bones and increases the likelihood of bone fractures.

Osteoporosis A bone disorder characterized by a reduction in bone mass, increased bone fragility, and an increased risk of fractures.

Overnutrition Poor nutritional status resulting from a dietary intake in excess of that which is optimal for health.

Oxalates Organic acids found in spinach, rhubarb, and other leafy green vegetables that can bind certain minerals and decrease their absorption.

Oxidative damage Damage caused by highly reactive oxygen molecules that steal electrons from other compounds, causing changes in structure and function.

Pancreas An organ that secretes digestive enzymes and bicarbonate ions into the small intestine during digestion.

Parathyroid hormone (PTH) A hormone secreted by the parathyroid gland that increases blood calcium levels.

Peak bone mass The maximum bone density attained at any time in life, usually occurring in young adulthood.

Pellagra The disease resulting from a deficiency of niacin.

Pepsin A protein-digesting enzyme produced by the stomach. It is secreted in the gastric juice in an inactive form and activated by acid in the stomach.

Peristalsis Coordinated muscular contractions that move food through the gastrointestinal tract.

pH A measure of acidity.

Phospholipid A type of fat that contains a phosphorus-containing group in addition to 2 fatty acids attached to a molecule of glycerol.

Phylloquinone The form of vitamin K found in plants.

Glossary

Phytate An inorganic phosphorus storage compound found in seeds and grains that can bind minerals and decrease their absorption.

Phytochemical A substance found in plant foods that is not an essential nutrient but may have health-promoting properties.

Polypeptide A chain of amino acids.

Polysaccharides Carbohydrates made up of many sugar units linked together.

Polyunsaturated fatty acid A fatty acid that contains two or more carbon-carbon double bonds.

Protein complementation Combining proteins from different sources so that they collectively provide the proportions of amino acids required to meet needs.

Protein-energy malnutrition (PEM) A condition characterized by wasting and an increased susceptibility to infection that results from the long-term consumption of insufficient energy and protein to meet needs.

Protein quality A measure of how efficiently a protein in the diet can be used to make body proteins.

Pyridoxine The chemical term for vitamin B_6.

Pyruvate A 3-carbon molecule produced during the breakdown of glucose in glycolysis.

Recommended Dietary Allowances (RDAs) Intakes recommended by the DRIs that are sufficient to meet the nutrient needs of almost all healthy people in a specific life-stage and gender group.

Refined Refers to foods that have undergone commercial processing that causes changes in various components of the original food.

Retinoids The chemical forms of preformed vitamin A: retinol, retinal, and retinoic acid.

Rhodopsin A light-sensitive compound found in the retina of the eye that is composed of the protein opsin loosely bound to retinal.

Rickets A vitamin D deficiency disease in children that is characterized by poor bone development because of inadequate calcium deposition.

Saliva A watery fluid produced and secreted into the mouth by the salivary glands. It contains lubricants, enzymes, and other substances.

Saturated fat or **fatty acid** A fatty acid in which the carbon atoms are bound to as many hydrogens as possible and which therefore contains no carbon-carbon double bonds.

Scurvy A vitamin C deficiency disease.

Simple carbohydrates Carbohydrates known as sugars that include monosaccharides and disaccharides.

Soluble fiber Fiber that either dissolves when placed in water or absorbs water. It includes pectins, gums, and some hemicelluloses.

Solutes Dissolved substances.

Solvent A fluid in which one or more substances dissolve.

Starch A carbohydrate made of many glucose molecules linked in straight or branching chains. The bonds that hold the glucose molecules together can be broken by the human digestive enzymes.

Sucrose A disaccharide formed by linking glucose to fructose. Sucrose, known as table sugar, is refined from sugarcane or sugar beets. It is the only sweetener that can be called "sugar" in the ingredient list on food labels in the United States.

Sugar The basic unit of carbohydrate. Only sucrose can be called "sugar" in the ingredient list on food labels.

Tannins Substances found in tea and some grains that can bind certain minerals and decrease their absorption.

Tocopherol The chemical name for vitamin E.

Tolerable Upper Intake Level (UL) The maximum daily intake that is unlikely to pose risks of adverse health effects to almost all individuals in the specified life-stage and gender group.

Trace elements Minerals required in the diet in amounts 100 mg or less per day or present in the body in amounts 0.01% of body weight or less.

Glossary

Trans fatty acid An unsaturated fatty acid in which the hydrogens are on opposite sides of the double bond.

Transferrin An iron transport protein in the blood.

Transit time The amount of time it takes food and waste products to move through the gastrointestinal tract.

Triglyceride (triacylglycerol) The major form of lipid in food and in the body. It consists of three fatty acids attached to a glycerol molecule.

Unsaturated fat or fatty acid A fatty acid that contains one or more carbon-carbon double bonds.

Urea A nitrogen-containing waste product that is excreted in the urine.

Vegan Referring to a pattern of food intake that eliminates all animal products.

Veins Vessels that carry blood toward the heart.

Very-low-density lipoproteins (VLDLs) Lipoproteins assembled by the liver that carry lipids from the liver and deliver triglycerides to body cells.

Vitamins Organic compounds needed in the diet in small amounts to promote and regulate the chemical reactions and processes needed for growth, reproduction, and maintenance of health.

Water-soluble vitamins Vitamins that dissolve in water.

Xerophthalmia A spectrum of eye conditions resulting from vitamin A deficiency that may lead to blindness. An early symptom is night blindness, and as deficiency continues, a lack of mucus leaves the eye dry and vulnerable to cracking and infection.

1. Institute of Medicine, Food and Nutrition Board. "Dietary Reference Intakes for Energy, Carbohydrates, Fiber, Fat, Protein, and Amino acids." Washington, D.C.: National Academy Press, 2002.

2. Wolraich, M. L., D. B. Wilson, and J. W. White. "The effect of sugar on behavior or cognition in children: a meta analysis." *Journal of the American Medical Association* 274 (1995): 1617–1618.

3. Salmeron, J., A. Ascherio, E.B. Rimm, et al. "Dietary fiber, glycemic load, and risk of NIDDM in men." *Diabetes Care* 20 (1997): 545–550.

4. USDA, Agricultural Service. "Results from USDA's 1994–1996 Continuing Survey of Food Intakes by Individuals and 1994–1996 Health Knowledge Survey." ARS Food Surveys Research Group, 1997. Available online at *http://www.barc.usda.gov/bhnrc/foodsurvey/home/htm.*

5. Marlett, J. A. "Sites and mechanisms for the hypocholesterolemic actions of soluble dietary fiber sources." *Fiber in Human Health and Disease*, eds. Kritevsky, D., and C. Bonfield. New York: Plenum Press, 1997, pp. 109–121.

6. Gerster, H. "The use of n-3 PUFAs (fish oil) in enteral nutrition." *International Journal for Vitamin and Nutrition Research* 65 (1995): 3–20.

7. Stone, N. J. "Fish consumption, fish oil, lipids, and coronary heart disease." *American Journal of Clinical Nutrition* 65 (1997): 1083–1086.

8. Messina, V. K., and K. I. Burke. "Position of the American Dietetic Association: vegetarian diets." *Journal of the American Dietetic Association* 97 (1997): 1317–1321.

9. Janelle, K. C., and S. I. Barr. "Nutrient intakes and eating behavior scores of vegetarian and nonvegetarian women." *Journal of the American Dietetic Association* 95 (1995): 180–189.

10. Walter, P. "Effects of vegetarian diets on aging and longevity." *Nutrition Reviews.* 55(II) (1997): S61–S68.

11. Askew, E.W. "Nutrition and performance in hot, cold, and high-altitude environments." *Nutrition in Exercise and Sport*, 3rd ed., ed. Wolinsky, I. Boca Raton, FL: CRC Press, 1998, pp. 597–619.

12. Shen, H.P. "Body fluids and water balance." *Biochemical and Physiological Aspects of Human Nutrition*, ed. Stipanuk, M. Philadelphia: W. B. Saunders, 2000, pp. 843–865.

13. Armstrong, L.E., and Y. Epstein. "Fluid-electrolyte balance during labor and exercise: concepts and misconceptions." *International Journal of Sport Nutrition* 9 (1999): 1–12.

14. Guyton J.R., M.A. Blazing, J. Hagar, et al. "Extended-release niacin vs. gemfibrozil for the treatment of low levels of high-density lipoprotein cholesterol. Niaspan-Gemfibrozil Study Group." *Archives of Internal Medicine* 160 (2000): 1177–1184.

References

15. Wyatt, K.M., P.W. Dimmock, P.W. Jones, P.M. Shaughn O'Brien. "Efficacy of vitamin B-6 in the treatment of premenstrual syndrome: systematic review." *British Medical Journal* 318 (1999): 1375–1381.

16. Honein, M., L. Paulozzi, T. Mathews, et al. "Impact of folic acid fortification in the US food supply on the occurrence of neural tube defects." *Journal of the American Medical Association* 285 (2001): 2981–2986.

17. Hemilä, H. "Vitamin C supplementation and common cold symptoms: Factors affecting the magnitude of the benefit." *Medical Hypotheses* 52 (1999): 171–178.

18. Maden, M. "Vitamin A in embryonic development." *Nutrition Reviews* 52 (1994): S3–S12.

19. Ross, D. A. "Vitamin A and public health." *Proceedings of the Nutrition Society* 57 (1998): 159–165.

20. Food and Nutrition Board, Institute of Medicine. "Dietary Reference Intakes: Vitamin A, Vitamin K, Arsenic, Boron, Chromium, Copper, Iodine, Iron, Manganese, Molybdenum, Nickel, Silicon, Vanadium, and Zinc." Washington, D.C.: National Academy Press, 2001.

21. Steiner, M. "Vitamin E, a modifier of platelet function: rationale and use in cardiovascular and cerebrovascular disease." *Nutrition Reviews* 57 (1999): 306–309.

22. New, S.A., S.P. Robins, M.K. Campbell, et al. "Dietary influences on bone mass and bone metabolism: further evidence of a positive link between fruit and vegetable consumption and bone health." *American Journal of Clinical Nutrition* 71 (2000): 142–151.

23. King, J. C., and C. L. Keen. "Zinc." *Modern Nutrition in Health and Disease*, 9th ed., eds. Shils, M. E., J. A. Olson, M. Shike, and A. C. Ross. Baltimore: Williams & Wilkins, 1999, pp. 223–239.

24. Uauy, R., M. Olivares, and M. Gonzales. "Essentiality of copper in humans." *American Journal of Clinical Nutrition* 67, supplement (1998): 952S–959S.

25. Xu, G. L., S. C. Wang, B. Q. Gu, et al. "Further investigation on the role of selenium deficiency in the aetiology and pathogenesis of Keshan disease." *Biomedical and Environmental Sciences* 10 (1997): 316–326.

26. Van der Haar, F. "The challenge of the global elimination of iodine deficiency disorders." *European Journal of Clinical Nutrition* 51, supplement (1997): S3–S8.

27. Furnee, C. A. "Prevention and control of iodine deficiency: a review of a study on the effectiveness of oral iodized oil in Malawi." *European Journal of Clinical Nutrition* 51, supplement (1998): S9–S10.

28. Lukaski, H. C. "Chromium as a supplement." *Annual Review of Nutrition* 19 (1999): 279–301.

29. American Dental Association. "Fluoridation facts." Available online at *http://www.ada.org/consumer/fluoride/facts/ff-menu.html*.

30. National Institutes of Health, National Heart, Lung, and Blood Institute. "Clinical guidelines on the identification, evaluation, and treatment of overweight and obesity in adults. Executive summary, June 1998." Available online at *http://www.nhlbi.nih.gov/guidelines/obesity/ob_home.htm*.

31. "Prevalence of Overweight and Obesity Among Adults: United States 1999–2000." Centers for Disease Control and Prevention. Available online at *http://www.cdc.gov/nchs/releases/02news/obesityonrise.htm.*

32. Young, L.R., M. Nestle. "The contribution of expanding portion sizes to the obesity epidemic." *American Journal of Public Health* 92 (2002): 246–249.

33. Hill, J.O., H.R. Wyatt, G.W. Reed, and J.C. Peters. "Obesity and the environment: Where do we go from here?" *Science* 299 (2003): 853–855.

Bibliography

American Dental Association. "Fluoridation facts." Available online at *http://www.ada.org/consumer/fluoride/facts/ff-menu.html.*

Armstrong, L.E., and Epstein, Y. "Fluid-electrolyte balance during labor and exercise: concepts and misconceptions." *International Journal of Sport Nutrition* 9 (1999): 1–12.

Askew, E.W. "Nutrition and performance in hot, cold, and high-altitude environments." *Nutrition in Exercise and Sport*, 3rd ed., ed. Wolinsky, I. Boca Raton, FL: CRC Press, 1998, pp. 597–619.

Collins MD, Mao GE. "Teratology of retinoids." *Annual Review of Pharmacology and Toxicology* 39 (1999): 399–430.

Furnee, C.A. "Prevention and control of iodine deficiency: a review of a study on the effectiveness of oral iodized oil in Malawi." *European Journal of Clinical Nutrition* 51, supplement (1998): S9–S10.

Gerster, H. "The use of n-3 PUFAs (fish oil) in enteral nutrition." *International Journal for Vitamin and Nutrition Research* 65 (1995): 3–20.

Guyton J.R., Blazing M.A., Hagar J., et al. "Extended-release niacin vs. gemfibrozil for the treatment of low levels of high-density lipoprotein cholesterol. Niaspan-Gemfibrozil Study Group." *Archives of Internal Medicine* 160 (2000): 1177–1184.

Hemilä, H. "Vitamin C supplementation and common cold symptoms: factors affecting the magnitude of the benefit." *Medical Hypotheses* 52 (1999): 171–178.

Hill, J.O., Wyatt, H.R., Reed, G.W., and Peters, J.C. "Obesity and the environment: where do we go from here?" *Science* 299 (2003): 853–855.

Honein, M., Paulozzi, L., Mathews, T., et al. "Impact of folic acid fortification in the US food supply on the occurrence of neural tube defects." *Journal of the American Medical Association* 285 (2001): 2981–2986.

Institute of Medicine, Food and Nutrition Board. "Dietary Reference Intakes for Energy, Carbohydrates, Fiber, Fat, Protein, and Amino acids." Washington D.C.: National Academy Press, 1999–2004. Available online at *http://www.nap.edu.*

Janelle, K.C., and Barr, S.I. "Nutrient intakes." *Journal of the American Dietetic Association* 95 (1995): 180–189.

King, J.C., and Keen, C.L. "Zinc." *Modern Nutrition in Health and Disease*, 9th ed., eds. Shils, M.E., Olson, J.A., Shike, M., and Ross, A.C. Baltimore: Williams & Wilkins, 1999, pp. 223–239.

Lukaski, H.C. "Chromium as a supplement." *Annual Review of Nutrition* 19 (1999): 279–301.

Maden, M. "Vitamin A in embryonic development." *Nutrition Reviews* 52 (1994): S3–S12.

Marlett, J.A. "Sites and mechanisms for the hypocholesterolemic actions of soluble dietary fiber sources." *Fiber in Human Health and Disease*, eds. Kritevsky, D., and Bonfield, C. New York: Plenum Press, 1997, pp. 109–121.

Messina, V.K., and Burke, K.I. "Position of the American Dietetic Association: Vegetarian diets." *Journal of the American Dietetic Association* 97 (1997): 1317–1321.

National Institutes of Health, National Heart, Lung, and Blood Institute. "Clinical guidelines on the identification, evaluation, and treatment of overweight and obesity in adults. Executive summary, June 1998." Available online at *http://www.nhlbi.nih.gov/guidelines/obesity/ob_home.htm*.

New, S.A., Robins, S.P., Campbell, M.K., et al. "Dietary influences on bone mass and bone metabolism: Further evidence of a positive link between fruit and vegetable consumption and bone health." *American Journal of Clinical Nutrition* 71 (2000): 142–151.

"Prevalence of Overweight and Obesity Among Adults: United States 1999–2000." Centers for Disease Control and Prevention. Available online at *http://www.cdc.gov/nchs/releases/02news/obesityonrise.htm*.

Ross, D.A. "Vitamin A and public health." *Proceedings of the Nutrition Society* 57 (1998): 159–165.

Salmeron, J., Ascherio, A., Rimm, E.B., et al. "Dietary fiber, glycemic load, and risk of NIDDM in men." *Diabetes Care* 20 (1997): 545–550.

Shen, H.P. "Body fluids and water balance." *Biochemical and Physiological Aspects of Human Nutrition*, ed. Stipanuk, M. Philadelphia: W.B. Saunders, 2000, pp. 843–865.

Steiner, M. "Vitamin E, a modifier of platelet function: Rationale and use in cardiovascular and cerebrovascular disease." *Nutrition Reviews* 57 (1999): 306–309.

Stone, N. J. "Fish consumption, fish oil, lipids, and coronary heart disease." *American Journal of Clinical Nutrition* 65 (1997): 1083–1086.

Bibliography

Uauy, R., Olivares, M., and Gonzales, M. "Essentiality of copper in humans." *American Journal of Clinical Nutrition* 67, supplement (1998): 952S–959S.

USDA, Agricultural Service. "Results from USDA's 1994–1996 Continuing Survey of Food Intakes by Individuals and 1994–1996 Health Knowledge Survey." ARS Food Surveys Research Group, 1997. Available online at *http://www.barc.usda.gov/bhnrc/foodsurvey /home/htm.*

Van der Haar, F. "The challenge of the global elimination of iodine deficiency disorders." *European Journal of Clinical Nutrition* 51, supplement (1997): S3–S8.

Walter, P. "Effects of vegetarian diets on aging and longevity." *Nutrition Reviews* 55(II) (1997): S61–S68.

Wolraich, M.L., Wilson, D.B., and White, J.W. "The effect of sugar on behavior or cognition in children: A meta analysis." *Journal of the American Medical Association* 274 (1995): 1617–1618.

Wyatt, K.M., Dimmock, P.W., Jones, P.W., Shaughn O'Brien, P.M. "Efficacy of vitamin B-6 in the treatment of premenstrual syndrome: Systematic review." *British Medical Journal* 318 (1999): 1375–1381.

Xu, G.L., Wang, S.C., Gu, B.Q., et al. "Further investigation on the role of selenium deficiency in the aetiology and pathogenesis of Keshan disease." *Biomedical and Environmental Sciences* 10 (1997): 316–326.

Young, L.R., and Nestle, M. "The contribution of expanding portion sizes to the obesity epidemic." *American Journal of Public Health* 92 (2002): 246–249.

Index

Cobalamin (vitamin B_{12}), 10, 95,
    159, 163
    absorption, 98
    deficiency of, 70–71, 96–98
    function, 96, 98, 109
    sources, 16–17, 97–98, 143
    water-soluble, 89, 109
Coenzyme, 90, 95, 98, 109, 131,
    159
Cofactor, 110, 120, 159
Collagen, 99, 159
Colon. *See* Intestine
Copper
    absorption, 112, 126
    deficiency, 126
    function, 126–127, 131
    need, 110
    sources, 126, 143
    toxicity, 126
Cretinism, 128–129, 159

Daily Value, 12, 19, 113, 159
DASH diet. *See* Dietary
    Approaches to Stop
    Hypertension diet
Dehydration, 82, 84
    death by, 78
    prevention, 77
    risk of, 83–84
    symptoms, 72, 81, 83, 85, 87
Diabetes mellitus, 54, 124, 159
    risk of, 10, 19, 27–28, 30–31,
        33, 39, 43, 53, 69, 130
Diet, 10, 158, 167
    American, 10, 15, 19, 21, 23,
        31–32, 40, 43, 55, 66, 70,
        92, 113, 116, 128, 133,
        144–145, 159
    carbohydrates in, 2, 7, 20–23,
        27, 30–33, 63, 132,
        141–142, 144
    fiber, 2, 34–35, 37–43, 54,
        132, 142, 157

healthy, 1–2, 6, 9, 11, 14–15,
    17, 19, 33, 57, 69, 71,
    132–133, 141–142, 144–145
lipids in, 2, 7, 46–47, 49–53,
    55–57, 63, 100, 103, 115,
    132, 141–142, 144
minerals, 2, 8, 110–113,
    115–122, 124–128,
    130–132, 143–144, 165
protein in, 2, 7–8, 51, 59–60,
    62–66, 70–71, 78, 94, 119,
    141–144, 164, 168–169
supplements, 2, 6, 10, 46, 62,
    66, 92, 94–98, 100, 103,
    106–108, 112–113, 119,
    121, 124–130, 143–145
vegetarian, 8, 66–71, 170
vitamins in, 2, 8, 88–90,
    92–94, 102, 104, 106, 108,
    119, 133, 143–144
water, 8, 74–75, 85
Dietary Approaches to Stop
    Hypertension (DASH) diet,
    115, 159
Dietary guidelines, 10, 15,
    18–19, 132, 141
Dietary Reference Intakes
    (DRIs), 9–10, 19, 31, 40, 55,
    66, 89, 111, 141, 156, 159, 168
Dietary Supplements Health and
    Education Act (1994), 2
Digestion, 4, 6, 134, 159, 161, 167
    of carbohydrates, 5, 7, 26, 39,
        164
    of fibers, 7, 17, 34–39, 43
    of lipids, 5, 7, 37–38, 50–51,
        157
    of proteins, 5, 60
Digestive system, 34, 161, 165,
    167, 169, *see also* Gastro-
    intestinal (GI) tract
    components, 4–5
    function, 4

Picture Credits

page:

5: Lambda Science Artwork
13: Courtesy of the NIH
14: © Peter Lamb
18: Courtesy USDA
22: © Jim Perkins
25: © Jim Perkins
29: © Jim Perkins
32: Photo by Keith Weller, Agricultural Research Service, USDA
36: Photo by Keith Weller, Agricultural Research Service, USDA
38: © Jim Perkins
45: © Jim Perkins
48: © Jim Perkins
61: © Jim Perkins
63: © Jim Perkins
65: (a) Associated Press, AP/ Suzanne Plunkett
65: (b) Associated Press, AP/ David Guttenfelder
82: © Jim Perkins
101: © Jim Perkins
105: © CORBIS
123: (a+b) © Gladden Willis/ Visuals Unlimited
129: © Earl & Nazima Kowell/ CORBIS
137: Courtesy CDC
140: Information from Journal of the American Medical Association

Frontis A: Photo by Peggy Greb, Agricultural Research Service, USDA
Frontis B: Photo by Scott Bauer, Agricultural Research Service, USDA